D0248916

A FAMILY HISTORY OF ILLNESS

a FAMILY HISTORY of ILLNESS

MEMORY AS MEDICINE

Brett L. Walker

A MCLELLAN BOOK

UNIVERSITY OF WASHINGTON PRESS
Seattle

A *Family History of Illness* was supported by a grant from the McLellan Endowment, established through the generosity of Martha McCleary McLellan and Mary McLellan Williams.

Copyright © 2018 by the University of Washington Press
Printed and bound in the United States of America
Design by Katrina Noble
Composed in Electra, typeface designed by William Addison Dwiggins

22 21 20 19 18   5 4 3 2 1

All rights reserved. No part of this publication may be reproduced or transmitted in any form or by any means, electronic or mechanical, including photocopy, recording, or any information storage or retrieval system, without permission in writing from the publisher.

UNIVERSITY OF WASHINGTON PRESS
www.washington.edu/uwpress

LIBRARY OF CONGRESS CATALOGING-IN-PUBLICATION DATA
Names: Walker, Brett L., 1967– author.
Title: A family history of illness : memory as medicine / Brett L. Walker.
Description: Seattle : University of Washington Press, 2018. | Includes
    bibliographical references and index. |
Identifiers: LCCN 2017028010 (print) | LCCN 2017031983 (ebook) |
    ISBN 9780295743042 (ebook) | ISBN 9780295743035 (hardcover :
    acid-free paper)
Subjects: LCSH: Walker, Brett L., 1967—Health. | Walker, Brett L., 1967—
    Family. | Walker, Brett L., 1967—Homes and haunts—Montana. |
    Immunologic diseases—Patients—United States—Biography. |
    Genetic disorders—Patients—United States—Biography. | Families—
    Psychological aspects. | History—Psychological aspects. | Memory—
    Psychological aspects. | Farm life—Montana. | Montana—Biography.
Classification: LCC CT275.W24518 (ebook) | LCC CT275.W24518 A3 2017
    (print) | DDC 920.009786—dc23
LC record available at https://lccn.loc.gov/2017028010

Photographs are from the author's collection, excepting those of Charles Janeway with microscope (p. 42; Boston Children's Hospital Archive, Collection MC7, Box 5, Folder 13), Charles Janeway protesting (p. 49; Boston Children's Hospital Archive, Collection MC7, Box 6, Folder 33), Ogden Carr Bruton (p. 81; National Archives photo 111-SC-32178), and the *Menace* newspaper (p. 157).

To my kin, who all immigrated to
the United States at some point . . .

CONTENTS

ACKNOWLEDGMENTS

This book started to take shape during a year spent teaching at Harvard University beginning in the fall of 2015. One evening, while dining with David Armitage, who chaired the Department of History at the time, I told him about the project and what I was trying to accomplish with it. I had struggled with how to narrate such a personal story, and how to make it intellectually substantive while still retaining the flavor of a memoir, and I floated some possible titles by him. While we sipped our beers, he took a pen from his bag and wrote A FAMILY HISTORY OF ILLNESS in large block letters on the paper tablecloth. "That's your title," he said. Indeed, that became the title, as well as the central theme of the book. I still have the piece of tablecloth, and now I have this book, in part because of David's support and suggestions.

I learned a great deal during my year in the Boston area, and I owe the opportunity to Ian Miller, my friend and colleague.

Harvard buzzed with intellectual energy, and my batteries needed recharging. I am indebted to both the Reischauer Institute for Japanese Studies, my principal sponsor at Harvard, and the Department of History, the academic home of the courses I taught, for making my visit possible. Ted Bestor, faculty director of the Reischauer Institute, and Stacie Matsumoto, the assistant director, also made my visit possible and saw to my every need, including a helpful research stipend.

On my return to Bozeman, colleagues, friends, and family read my fledgling manuscript and offered valuable insights. LaTrelle Scherffius, my wife and partner, read an early draft of the manuscript and offered many important editorial suggestions and inspirational support, as did my father, Nelson Walker. My mother, Linda Walker, gave endless support and watched the Reese Creek home front while we lived in Cambridge. My stepson and a philosopher, Andrew Scherffius, taught me how to interpret Heidegger's *Being and Time*, which was no small task. My colleague Michael Reidy read the entire manuscript and offered a lively critical assessment, as did my colleague Dale Martin. Tim LeCain allowed early access to the manuscript of his forthcoming book, *The Matter of History*. Gregg Mitman read the manuscript for the press and transformed the book with his smart suggestions. Kirk Branch delivered enthusiastically a pronouncement or two about adverbs. Julie Van Pelt at UW Press offered many effective suggestions. I also received helpful comments from an anonymous reader for the press. At Montana State University, I receive generous support for my research program from Nic Rae, dean of the College of Letters and Science, and Renee Reijo Pera, the vice president for research and economic development. Scott Smiley did the outstanding index.

This book would not have been possible without the support of Harvard University's Countway Library of Medicine and the Houghton Library, as well as the Boston Children's Hospital Archive, the Massachusetts Historical Society in Boston, the Montana Historical Society in Helena, Montana State University's Renne Library, and Princeton University's Registrar's Office. A Guggenheim Fellowship funded some of this research. I appreciate the patience that my ninety-five-year-old grandmother, Frances Dwyer, exhibited while I recorded our many conversations about my Montana family's history, usually at Taco Treat. I also grilled my parents and other family members about family-related questions for years as I gathered information for this project, including quizzing my brother, Aaron, about his memories. I discovered aspects of my family history during this project that proved a little jarring, but everybody kept a brave face.

Many people supported me and nurtured me as I recovered in the months after my hospitalization in 2010–11, and I will always be grateful to them, particularly Christine Marran and Ben Swartz. I'll always remember the heroic efforts of the team at the University of Minnesota's Health Center, including those of my doctor Greg Vercellotti. I am indebted to the nurses at the Bozeman Health Cancer Center, where I receive my monthly infusions, and to my doctor in Bozeman, Luke Omohundro. Ash's Okinawan Karate was a gem, and I owe Lisa and Brian a debt of gratitude for keeping me disciplined and healthy. Mostly, my deepest appreciation goes to my parents and brother, Linda, Nelson, and Aaron, and to LaTrelle, Liz, Andrew, Wayne, May, Fiona, and Simona, for being my family.

A FAMILY HISTORY OF ILLNESS

Nightmares

I AWOKE STARTLED AND FEVERISH. "WHERE AM I?" I thought. The back of my head pounded. I was thirsty and drenched in sweat. When I coughed, the pounding intensified and ripped along the center of my scalp toward my forehead, piercing a point between my eyes. A white hospital gown clung to my shivering body. The vision in my right eye became blurrier the more I hacked. My neck and shoulders tensed as I turned my head to look out a window near the bed—I saw only the inky black of the night sky.

I lifted myself upright to get a better view, and the sweaty hospital gown tightened around my shoulders, the fabric constraining me and chafing against my skin. I could feel tape tugging at the hairs on my arms and face, tying me to clear plastic hoses. I vaguely remembered that these tubes were important: they tethered me to rhythmic pumps and spherical tanks that kept me alive. I raised my body a little higher and, turning my head again, peered out the window, looking for clues to my whereabouts.

I saw no answers outside. Instead, I saw only a partly transparent reflection of my gaunt face, gauzy and ashen in the dim green light of some small, medical-looking machine. I adjusted my head to block the light and looked outside, through my ghostly face. Below me, floodlights lit a multistory parking structure, and a blizzard swirled in the light. The gusting winds came off a nearby frozen river. The snow, illuminated in the conical beams projected by the floodlights, made brilliant white streaks before vanishing into the cover of darkness. I was momentarily hypnotized, swept away in thought.

The floodlights came to represent the present, and the surrounding darkness the poorly lit past—where the snow had come from and where it was going, into an unknown future. The night was in rapid motion, obeying wind and weather— nothing stays in the present for long. Seeing all that snow outside, I felt it would kill me in seconds should I enter it. "I dreaded the cold much more than the enemy"—George Orwell's words, about his overriding fear while in the trenches of Alcubierre, floated through my head. "I had even lain awake at nights thinking of the cold," he said. I was also awake at night thinking of the cold, and it frightened me, too.

As my consciousness came back into the room, I heard the slow rhythm of the intravenous pump. I saw that the green light that filled the room came from an electrocardiographic machine. Then I saw a thin crack of light emanating from a bathroom, the door of which stood slightly ajar. "I'm in a hospital," I thought. "But what hospital?" There was a woman in the bathroom. A chill shot up my spine, making me shake violently again. I was flooded by feelings of anxiety. "What are you fucking doing?" I shouted. "You're watching me!" I heard something drop to the floor. It sounded like a heavy book, its pages fanning noisily as it hit the floor. I became uncontrollably paranoid. I wanted to escape, but the damp gown, tape, and plastic hoses restrained me. "What the hell is going on in here?" I demanded. "Let me the fuck out of here!"

The bathroom door swung open and, fumbling with her glasses, a startled woman emerged from the lit room. Almost simultaneously, another door swung open, florescent lights burst on, and a large male nurse entered, his eyes darting about, looking for the source of the commotion. The light flooded over me like a bucket of cold water and I began to remember. I was in a drug-induced delirium, likely from large amounts of Demerol pulsing through my veins. I was at the University of Minnesota Medical Center dying of an unstoppable case of pneumonia and pleural effusion (fluid between tissues that line the chest and lungs). The entire hallucination of snow and cold and time slipped away, dreamlike in how it came and went—as I write now, I can retrieve only fragments of it. The harsh fluorescent lights shone accusingly on my shivering body. Embarrassed, I could only muster a timid "I'm cold." I was not doing well and I knew it.

— · —

Five days before, I had been admitted to the University of Minnesota emergency room after an urgent-care doctor in Minneapolis refused to refill my antibiotics for pneumonia. "It's against policy," he explained in a heavy Indian accent. "If these antibiotics don't work the first time, you need to go to the hospital immediately." It was sound medical advice, given that I could barely walk on my own. Draped over my girlfriend's shoulders, I slowly made my way across the road to the emergency room and was immediately admitted. A swarm of doctors, nurses, and medical students descended on my clammy body, poking, prodding, and taking chest x-rays. They then began talking among themselves, just out of earshot.

When they returned to my bedside, a middle-aged doctor stepped forward from the group and said I was in serious trouble. I needed to be moved to the University of Minnesota's main hospital as soon as the paperwork could be completed. I was in a daze, but I managed to say, "Sounds good, I guess." While I was being loaded into an ambulance for transfer, the same doctor leaned over my gurney and asked, "Have you gotten a tattoo recently?" I shook my head no. "Are you sexually active?" I just stared at him, a little shy about the question. Then he asked, "Do you have a family history of illness?" I kept staring at him. "A family history of illness," I whispered back at him, my dry lips wrapping around the words as they slowly dissipated into the crowd of doctors and nurses. Little did I know then how many times I'd hear this question during my prolonged stay in the hospital, or how it would echo into my life even after my eventual recovery.

Then I was lifted into the ambulance. The doors closed behind me, the painkillers took over, and everything became less urgent. Through the windows, I watched reflections of red emergency lights flashing against the glass office buildings we drove past. The siren was deafening. "This is all because of me," I thought. I had never been in an ambulance before.

Once at the hospital, I was transported to a series of rooms, each more specialized and secluded than the last, each emblematic, in my delirium, of my deteriorating medical condition, as if I were spiraling down through Dante's concentric circles of hell. I started out in a room with a television that buzzed with CNN and news of the shooting of Arizona representative Gabrielle Giffords. I was soon moved to the inner sanctum, where the mechanical pumping of advanced medical technologies replaced twenty-four-hour news coverage. I felt like I was on the bridge of a galaxy-class starship.

My pneumonia continued to worsen, however, and I ended up in the ICU with pleural effusion. Eventually, a hole drilled in my chest allowed a hose to be threaded in that continuously pumped a thick yellow fluid out of my lungs, to keep me breathing. At first, a medical student had tried to insert the plastic hose, but when she stumbled a third and then fourth time, the observing doctor, a no-nonsense woman, ran out of patience and took the hose herself and forcefully threaded it into my chest, explaining the process to the student. As a teacher myself, I admired her cool pedagogical acumen: I felt I could probably perform the procedure in a pinch, had I not been so high on painkillers. Later, as I slowly recovered, I carried the pump with me like a briefcase, its electric motor humming and its holding tank always full. "How could there possibly be any more of this putrid yellow shit in my body?" I wondered more than once. But the pump sucked it out for days. If the gelatinous fluid was not removed, it could cause problems later, after it hardened— but only if I first survived the pneumonia. Periodically, I was injected with anticoagulants, which broke up the hardening fluid so the machine could suck it out.

Despite all the interventions, the pneumonia only spread and got worse. My heart rate spiked and I was in excruciating pain from coughing despite liberal doses of Demerol—my ribs bruised badly. One nurse tried to calm me by recounting his own successful fight with pneumonia. I liked him: it soothed me to think that somebody else had suffered through this nightmare and had ultimately survived. But I didn't stay with this nurse for long. I didn't stay with any of them for long. I descended deeper and deeper into the hospital—moving closer to the morgue, I suspected. "Less distance to transport me in the end," I thought. While in the ICU, I overheard one of my pulmonologists recommend that my mother and father be contacted. I was dying and my parents needed to be brought to my bedside while I was still conscious. "Christ, I'm forty-four," I whispered to a nearby nurse. She looked back sympathetically.

When I heard about my impending death, my life didn't begin to flash before my eyes in what is, I've been told, the customary manner. Instead, my family history of illness began to flow by in bits and pieces. I couldn't remember anyone in my family having had pneumonia, but I had never asked about family members' health in any detail. My mother had nearly died from hepatitis as a little girl—I knew that. But that hardly seemed related to my killer pneumonia. Bodies and health weren't really topics in my family. Rather, our stories were about the world outside, about hunting, fishing, skiing, and farming. Still, my doctors urgently wanted to talk about bodily stories. I'm not sure I knew any.

As my mother made her way from Washington State to Minnesota, my lungs continued to fill with fluid. Bag after plastic bag of powerful antibiotics failed to help, and the infection kept spreading. The pump in my chest could barely keep up, and my heart hammered at 140 beats per minute. I heard the conversation about contacting my parents, but thinking about my own death was like swimming in room-temperature gravy. My mind was all over the place: I had been sick before but had always recovered. I had always gotten better. At some point, however, it started to dawn on me that I was not going to recover this time. My life would end at forty-four in the Twin Cities of Minneapolis and Saint Paul. As a child of the West Coast, I was not even sure I could identify Minnesota on a map, and I was going to die there.

— · —

I had traveled to Minneapolis that winter to visit my new girl-friend, a fellow academic. We had met at the University of Minnesota's Twin Cities campus months earlier when I was there to lecture. Now, in late December, we planned to fly from Minneapolis to Portland, Oregon, near where we both had grown up. The morning we were to depart, I woke with a debilitating fever. I could barely move. I managed to board the plane, but once in Portland I immediately visited an urgent-care doctor. After a chest x-ray, he determined that I had early signs of pneumonia and he gave me antibiotics. At first they worked, if slowly, and I recovered somewhat, but then my condition started to worsen once more. By the time my girlfriend and I returned to Minneapolis, my health was slipping away from me. By New Year's Eve, I could only lie in bed and sweat, my head pounding. The next day, we visited the Minneapolis urgent-care clinic.

The day before my mother arrived in Minneapolis, doctors from the University of Minnesota's immunology department got involved in my case. One of them, a strikingly handsome research professor, had both my mother and my girlfriend completely smitten. He could have told them to put me down and they probably would have pulled the plug. He called for more elaborate blood testing because he couldn't understand how they were losing an otherwise healthy forty-four-year-old man. In Montana, I had regularly competed in Bridger Bowl community ski races, and I had raced mountain bikes throughout the Pacific Northwest. I was in excellent cardiovascular health. In fact, my attending physician later told me, "Had you not been in such good health, you never would've made it." One late afternoon, when I was alone, the handsome professor came into my room and looked at the bedside charts, his back to me. Then he came to my bed and said in a soft voice: "I think I know what's wrong with you, Brett." As he started to walk out of the room, he stopped, faced me, and asked, "By the way, I need to know: do you have a family history of illness?" I just stared at him. I was eager to hear his diagnosis.

The immunology department had hit upon a lifesaving breakthrough: through the more elaborate blood tests, doctors discovered that my immunoglobulins—particularly my gamma globulins—were virtually nonexistent, and they ordered an immediate infusion of human immunoglobulins. Immuno-globulins are glycoprotein molecules produced by white blood cells that serve as antibodies to fight bacterial infections, such as the one attacking my lungs. I had the white blood cells, but for some unknown reason my body had stopped produc-ing immunoglobulins. At first, doctors suspected this absence might be symptomatic of blood cancer, or perhaps lymphoma. But a battery of tests revealed that I did not have lymphoma, even though I had a significantly heightened risk of it, along with a risk of gastrointestinal cancers. My doctors finally diag-nosed me with the misleadingly benign-sounding condition of common variable immunodeficiency (CVID). This meant nothing to me at the time. But I quickly learned that it isn't common and is anything but benign.

What happened next, in probably the deepest moment of my Demerol-induced haze, was a kind African American nurse hanging a bag of immunoglobulins on my IV stand and saying, "There's magic in this bag. I've seen it before. You'll be just fine now." She then wiped my forehead with a damp towel and, turning her back to me, started keying information into the IV pump. She was one of many medical personnel who dramat-ically entered and exited my life at the hospital, almost like angels. Within minutes, I went into rigors, a violent convulsive shaking caused by introduction of the new medication: it is one of several possible side effects, none of which are pleasant. A chill started deep in my lower spine, beginning as a pinprick and then spreading outward until my whole body was convulsing. I had never been so cold. I shook ferociously, and the nurse and my girlfriend piled on top of me to try to warm me and keep me from shaking. Someone immediately reduced the drip speed, and the chill slowly receded and I fell asleep. I have no idea how long I slept, but after I woke I never allowed another drop of Demerol in my veins—I am convinced that the drug made me hallucinate on several occasions. My fever began to subside. The immunoglobulins had worked.

With repeated treatments, I steadily improved. Even though my body remained weak and vulnerable, all I wanted to do was leave the hospital. If that meant walking up and down the halls, taking my IV bag and chest pump for thrice-daily walks, then that's what I did. It also meant peeing and shitting on my own, which I also managed to accomplish and then boast to nurses about, like a grinning two-year-old. Every time a nurse or doctor entered my room, I managed an impish smile and told him or her how much better I felt, even if half the time I wasn't so sure. The night sweats in fact persisted for weeks, even after I left the hospital. After my discharge, I stayed in Minneapolis and spent a great deal of time at the Masonic Cancer Center getting monthly infusions of immunoglobulins, and I began to make a good recovery. My fitness regimen at the YWCA also helped, as did resigning as department chair, taking an overdue sabbatical, and teaching a couple of courses at the University of Minnesota. The infusions gave me what my body no longer produced, providing a vibrant immunity that kept me alive. My health held, but my relationship with my girlfriend did not, and I returned to Bozeman and my job at Montana State University in 2012.

— · —

My two weeks in the hospital were the most dangerous and destabilizing two weeks of my life, and they forever changed me. Frankly, I believe I have met the disease that will eventually kill me. My struggle with CVID, however, is not the subject of this book. In truth, such a story might prove overly familiar to many readers, another personal confrontation with illness similar to what millions of people face every day. Instead, this book is about the importance of history in understanding our bodies and, more broadly, our shared world. It presents a philosophy of history that integrates the body, memory, and immunity with the past and present—my effort to contextualize my experience with this immunological disorder within my story and my family's story to determine if I inherited CVID or acquired it as an adult.

The typical symptoms of CVID include chronic bacterial infections in the respiratory and gastrointestinal systems, so this book naturally explores the relationship between selfhood, history, and the communities of microorganisms that inhabit our bodies. It is not just about the microbiome's existence in our bodies but also about how those microbes may drive behavior and physiological development in a manner that destabilizes our understanding of the autonomy of selfhood. Science writer Ed Yong said of these microbial multitudes: "They guide the construction of our bodies, releasing molecules and signals that steer the growth of our organs. They educate our immune system, teaching it to tell friend from foe. They affect the development of the nervous system, and perhaps even influence our behavior. They contribute to our lives in profound and wide-ranging ways; no corner of our biology is untouched." Yong concluded, "If we ignore them, we are looking at our lives through a keyhole." I didn't want to write a keyhole-sized history. But all this talk about bugs and behavior begs the question:

to what degree do the microbes in our bodies influence our physiological development and behavior and, likewise, to what degree have they influenced important historical figures?

This book is also about how life experiences and expo-sures—our life histories, or those of our parents or grandpar-ents—become imprinted on the body's genome, expressing some genes while blocking others in life's epigenetic crapshoot, determining what person we ultimately become. If genetics defines the spectrum of the possible selves we might be, the incipient ones we inherit from our families, then it is our histo-ries, or lifetime experiences and exposures, that determine the selves that we in fact are—the phenotypes, or individuals result-ing from the interaction of genes and the environment. Here is another pertinent question: to what degree can historical expe-riences be inscribed on our genes and then made heritable to future generations, much as a ceramicist's carving tool etches patterns into clay?

This book investigates strikingly expanded and reduced scales of historical analysis, including something as small as a protein, the core building-block of life. Both the immunoglob-ulins that fight bodily intruders and the neurons that form the architecture of our brains are proteins—our memories, though they seem like old film reels rapidly clicking away in our minds, are built from such proteins, as is the immune system. There is a critical relationship between memory and health—mem-ory B-cells remain among the most powerful weapons in the immune system's arsenal; they rely on remembering past anti-gens to fight them—and this book explores how we remember, both immunologically and neurologically, and the reliability of those memories in relation to history. It postulates that his-torians serve as society's B-cells, and the archive as the cultural extension of the physiological neuronal forest that underlies our ability to remember and grow beyond the natural lifespan of the human brain. Throughout this book, I probe the authenticity of memory and how memory is drafted, often reluctantly, into the ranks of what becomes historical narrative, in all its diverse forms. This question frequently nags at me: Is the enterprise of history a cultural reflection of the biological necessity to remember?

Finally, this book explores the experiences of my family and the disease challenges they faced in order to make my life possible. It is about local threats to life, such as contagious disease outbreaks in colonial New England, and global ones, such as the eruption of Mount Tambora in 1815, which caused the "year without a summer" and killed millions around the world. It is about memory and the health and bodily scenes I witnessed as a child, including potent ones of my dying grandfather. It is about family stories and the continuation of life in the face of relentless bacterial and viral onslaught. It is about survival in a time before the 1928 invention of penicillin and the triumphant act of reproducing offspring before disease killed parents. I have been forced to ask: to what degree does context, family or otherwise, rather than our own individual effort, determine the person we ultimately become?

If in genetics the "hologenome" represents the collective genomic content of a host body and its microorganisms, a potent new way to view the holistic content of the body, then this book might be seen as a "holo-history," a narrative that transcends common scales and destabilizes the notion of autonomous selfhood in order to tell my body's story. It is about how the world outside me influenced who I am, as well as about how the world inside me influenced who I am. This book positions the body as history, and memory as medicine.

CHAPTER 1

Memories

WHEN MY PHYSICIANS ASKED, "DO YOU HAVE A FAMILY history of illness?" I remember thinking, "What does that even mean?" I could have told them truckloads about Japanese state building in the seventeenth century, or the causes of global environmental calamities in the twentieth — but virtually nothing about my family's history. It was a hell of a question to ask a historian in the midst of a pulsing fever and Demerol-induced fog. "How are such categories as family, history, and illness even connected?" I remember thinking later. The idea that words serve as historical categories was on the mind of Joan W. Scott in her famous 1986 article on gender when she explained, "Words, like the ideas and things they are meant to signify, have a history." Each one of these words — *family, history, illness* — is historically contingent and culturally meaningful, and a skilled historian could spend pages carefully unpacking the histories and meanings they have had as they have changed over time

and even across cultures. Yet my diseased body hardly felt like
a cultural signifier or emblematic of historical contexts: there
must be some real physical experience that transcends such
contingencies, some physical, unimagined structure on which
we can hang our stories.

During my hospitalization, as I inched closer to death, I
became almost obsessed with the question "Do you have a family history of illness?" It turns out, the question of family history
and illness is related to a field called narrative medicine, an
attempt by some doctors to better understand medical conditions
through clinical and symptomatic histories of both patients and
their families. In narrative medicine, patients become people
with stories rather than temporally static, historyless objects with
symptoms. Practitioners of narrative medicine seek to understand the psychological and personal history of the patient to
better understand illness, in an attempt to humanize medicine,
because nothing is more fundamentally human than stories. As
historian William Cronon observed, "Narrative remains essential to our understanding of history and the human place in
nature," adding that storytelling serves as our "best and most
compelling tool for searching out meaning in a conflicted and
contradictory world." Indeed, freestanding medical events — a
cold here or an infection there, for example — explain little, but
these medical events placed in careful causal relationship to
one another, and then contextualized historically and in family
patterns, have the ability to explain a great deal, particularly
about chronic disorders. "I always wanted to get people's stories
and access to their lives," wrote Oliver Sacks, an early advocate
of narrative medicine. "I feel I'm at the interface of biography
and biology, person and person-hood."

Historians, too, focus on accessing peoples' lives, but often
to tell bigger stories. By means of careful research and writing,

historians aim to give meaning to our world with rich contextualization and empirically based narratives; and these narratives,
when about our bodies and our families' health, can be a critical
part of understanding our own health. The idea that a chronic
health challenge can be understood exclusively through diagnosis in the present—the same elusive present of the snow temporarily illuminated in that conical beam of light beneath my
hospital window—hardly makes sense, given the complexities
of the body's interactions with the world. This holds true in
chronic social and national challenges, too. The historically
created world flows through our porous bodies every day. History is critical to understanding the past, present, and future,
particularly when it comes to understanding our bodies—and
therefore, memory can serve as a kind of medicine.

To interrogate the idea of a family history of illness conjures
other questions as well. If a family has a history, then what is
history? Does history encompass such topics as bodies or, even
more specifically, proteins, immune systems, neuronal forests,
and the bugs in our guts? What are the benefits and limitations
of history in understanding personal health troubles? More
important still, what role does history play in remedying the
serious challenges our fragile planet Earth faces? Does history
even have a place in a world so overwhelmingly dominated by
myopic fixation on satisfaction in the here and now? Do we
live in a world where history matters? I think it does, and in
the pages ahead, I will explain why; and contextualizing illness
within a person's life is a good place to start.

Right now, as I write, millions of people—some old, some
young, of every shape, size, color, and nationality—are being
diagnosed with life-threatening illnesses, many of which have
concrete family roots. Still other people are fighting deadly
diseases with powerful medicines, which represent doctors'

mobilizing centuries' worth of medical techniques and technologies to prolong and improve lives. Medicine, too, is built by
history, and facets of medical history stitch this book together—
as we'll see, the immunoglobulin therapy that saved me is the
product of an international accumulation of medical knowledge about blood. The threat of dying from disease is a very real
prospect for many throughout the world, as it always has been.
In colonial America, dying from smallpox, measles, typhus, or
any of scores of other dangerous diseases was common, probably so common that it was considered naturally caused and
thus rarely recorded. Disease, then, does not distinguish my
experience from that of others, or my family's experience from
that of other families. Rather, my fight with pneumonia and my
diagnosis with CVID have been a unifying experience, introducing me to a community of afflicted souls, many of them
wandering through historical documents. My CVID diagnosis
not only taught me the power of modern medicine but also
brought home the reality of "being mortal," in the words of
noted public health researcher Atul Gawande. I have come to
see this as a bedrock truth from which all history springs. In
the end, we all die, as our ancestors have; and many of us will
get seriously sick and die from some diagnosable and probably
painful illness. This has always been the case—disease is part of
life and part of history.

In 2013 and 2014, according to the Centers for Disease Control and Prevention, life expectancy in the United States stabi-
lized at 78.8 years, an astonishing number really, with just over
2.5 million people dying in 2013. Adjusted for age, this translates
to a little over 730 deaths per 100,000 US citizens in 2013, and
just under 725 deaths in 2014. For both 2013 and 2014, the leading killers were heart disease, malignant neoplasms or cancers,
chronic lower respiratory diseases, accidents, cerebrovascular

disease or strokes, Alzheimer's disease, diabetes, influenza and pneumonia, kidney disease, and suicide. Nearly 12 percent of people in the United States have heart disease, and one in every four deaths will result from it. The top killer cancers are cancer of the prostate; lung and bronchus; colon and rectum; corpus and uterus; urinary bladder, kidney and renal pelvis; thyroid; female breast cancer; skin melanomas; and non-Hodgkin's lymphoma. In the history of what has killed Americans, some things have remained remarkably stable. Heart disease and cancer, for example, have been the principal sources of death in the United States for the past seventy-five years.

Additionally, the National Institutes of Health estimate that nearly 24 million people in the United States struggle with one of eighty different autoimmune disorders, including such well-known ones as diabetes, rheumatoid arthritis, lupus, and inflammatory bowel disease. These autoimmune diseases are a strain on public health systems and have become the second leading cause of chronic illness in the United States. While 2.2 million women live with breast cancer, for example, 9.8 million women struggle with one of seven common autoimmune diseases, which decrease life expectancy by as much as fifteen years. In their brief history of autoimmunity, historians Warwick Anderson and Ian R. Mackay observe that autoimmune diseases "cause persistent suffering, following a drawn-out, often life-long, pattern of remission and recurrence, of control and exacerbation. Together they represent a major disease burden—and a rapidly growing global health problem, as the number of cases is increasing, for reasons still unclear." Even though scientists have studied the body's immune defenses since the nineteenth century, medical researchers coined the term *autoimmunity* only in 1957. But, following autoimmunity's recognition, they began devoting sustained attention to the immune system's "defensive contrivances turning rogue, going on the offensive against [a person's] own body."

Conversely, primary immunodeficiency diseases such as CVID are not nearly as prevalent as autoimmune disorders; but they are not as rare as one might think. One 2007 study found that among ten thousand households surveyed, doctors diagnosed twenty-three household members in eighteen households with immunodeficiency, including CVID. These results suggest that in the Unites States, one in twelve hundred people has primary immunodeficiency disease, or about 0.0833 percent of the population. Whether a person is dealing with a common killer such as cancer, or a more rare one such as CVID, struggle with a serious illness is a deeply human confrontation with the inevitable truth of one's finitude.

Paul Kalanithi, a thirty-seven-year-old neurosurgeon, was one such person diagnosed with a common killer and forced to prematurely confront his finitude. As death approached, he wrote about his struggle with lung cancer, a story later published as *When Breath Becomes Air*. It is in medical situations—a conversation with a doctor over an MRI of your lungs, for example, or over flagged blood test results—where most people initially confront their mortality. We first discuss our mortality, not with someone in priestly garb or a beloved family member, but with lab-coated doctors. Before his cancer diagnosis, Kalanithi, while talking with his own patients, realized this fact: "Questions intersecting life, death, and meaning, questions that all people face at some point, usually arise in a medical context." During one of these conversations, with a woman who had a brain tumor, Kalanithi began to see the "vastness of the chasm between the life she'd had last week and the one she was about to enter." As a physician, Kalanithi was less often "death's enemy," a vanquisher of disease, than "death's ambassador." Certainly, questions regarding my own mortality arose in such a medical context, with lab-coated doctors in a university hospital. They were the ones who asked me, "Do you have a family history of illness?" But historians, too, deal in death, because they dwell in a world inhabited by heroes and ghosts, many of whom are awoken from their eternal sleep to explain predicaments in the present.

Importantly, most of the major US killers, including lung cancer, can have serious hereditary elements and are therefore better understood in historical context. They are as much about blood as they are about other risk factors, such as lifestyle and environment. According to the American Heart Association, both heart disease and stroke are linked to family history. As are many forms of cancer, explains the American Cancer Society. In fact, most of the top ten diseases that kill people in the United States can be better understood through family histories. This manner of thinking historically about disease in the present is what interests me and what motivated me to write this book.

Historian Naomi Oreskes has written, "What matters to us about the past has everything to do with who we are, where we live, and what we think is important—to us, here and now, in the present." I couldn't agree more. Indeed, the motivations of historians, despite what they might claim in pursuit of the noble dream of objectivity, are inescapably about the present. My diagnosis with CVID has everything to do with my reevaluation of history in the pages of this book, and it ultimately led to my belief in history's irreplaceable role in understanding our selves and our world. If, as Oreskes observes of historians, "hiding our motivations hamstrings us intellectually and stylistically, isolates us from potential audiences, and undermines our ability to speak persuasively about the value of [our] work," then this book represents an embrace of the present—my diseased, bodily present, to be precise—in order to explore the mechanics of the past. And it all starts with personal memories, the ones that flooded my head while I recovered in the hospital.

— . —

I remember that, when I was a young boy, in the early summer of 1976, my family dismantled a Quonset hut in Great Falls, Montana, in order to move it to our wheat and barley farm near Cascade, about thirty minutes south. Cascade is a small town tucked along the Missouri River. On the west side of the river, where the town is situated, grassy hills and laccolithic buttes span northwest to the horizon until they run hard up against the Bob Marshall Wilderness and Glacier National Park. The east side is predominantly low-lying grasslands and cottonwood groves that comprise the Chestnut Valley, which extends to the Big Belt Mountains. Cascade sits in a transitional landscape, where the Missouri leaves behind its deeply carved breccia and conglomerate rocky gashes in the Adel Mountains Volcanic Field, near places like Wolf Creek and Craig, and slowly enters the vast expanse of rolling prairie near Great Falls, which extends north beyond the Hi-Line into southern Canada. The most prominent human-made feature in Cascade is the large grain elevator, around which the entire town orbits, and for good reason. Cascade is surrounded by good farm and ranch land, particularly on the east side of the Missouri.

"Unless everything in a man's memory of childhood is misleading," wrote Wallace Stegner in his memoir of his early years in the Hi-Line prairie, "there is a time somewhere between the ages of five and twelve which corresponds to the phase ethologists have isolated in the development of birds, when an impression lasting only a few seconds may be imprinted on the young bird for life." The memory of dismantling the Quonset hut with my grandfather made just such an impression on my birdlike memory. I was working at the Quonset with my grandfather, cleaning out old hunting paraphernalia, farm supplies, construction equipment, and other relics from his past businesses. I picked through every piece of wood and farm equipment, anticipating the mouse nests that, with squirming little hairless pink inhabitants, lay underneath. Old tractors, combine heads, rusty sickles, dead pickup trucks, and other large equipment served as my playground in those days. My grandfather, for my borderline useless efforts, paid me: this particular summer, I used my earnings to buy a lever-action Daisy BB gun, which I'd coveted for years. The BB gun became one of my favorite possessions. On the farm, I routinely patrolled the fields shooting at just about everything that meandered into my iron sights.

I was the only grandchild in our family that my grandfather knew well, simply by virtue of my age. I relished working with him—I must have been a complete pest. I wanted to be a farmer so badly it ached. He was my guide. He was my future. I would beg to ride in his pickup when we were at the Cascade farm. Like his black lab, Queen, I watched his every movement around the farmhouse, waiting for some evidence that he was heading out into the fields. "Dad, just take him," my mother pleaded. He always kept an old Sears and Roebuck bolt-action .22 in the truck, its barrel pointed toward the floor. He and I shot gophers with it: he complained that they destroyed crops and damaged farm equipment. To me the reason hardly mattered. Being a little farm boy, I thought shooting at gophers with my grandfather was about as much fun as a human being could possibly have in this world. "You know, Dad adored you," my mother once told me. I adored him, too.

That summer day when we cleaned the Quonset, my mother told me before I left to help: "Watch Grandpa. He's not supposed to be smoking. He's very sick from smoking, Brett." At the time, my grandfather was on the early side of his midfifties. In his youth, and up through his time in the air force until about 1967, he had been a powerful man, but as he entered his fifties his health had failed. First diabetes dogged him, and now lung cancer did. After working for a half hour packing boxes and moving farm equipment, he would have a smoke, as he always did, while sitting on the tailgate of his truck or leaning against a tractor. He rarely spoke when he smoked; he either looked to the ground, carefully pushing rocks or dirt with the tip of his boot, or looked off into the distance. I knew only this quiet side of him. I remember him sitting at the kitchen table at the Great Falls house, for example, smoking a cigarette, calling a plumber or electrician, and stroking Dusty, his cat, who sprawled on his lap. Even in these trivial acts he seemed like a superman to me; the cat, on the other hand, was a vile, hateful creature that tolerated nobody but him.

LeRoy Belote, my grandfather, was a quiet man, and he was comfortable in his silence. I suspect he hoped other people were comfortable with it too. I imagine he felt at home with the man he was; he did not require constant movement and noise, the clumsy impulse to ripple an otherwise clear reflection on water. That kind of clarity can expose aspects of a person's life one would rather not confront. It's like a fly-fishing line on the glassy stretch of the Missouri that glides through Cascade, where we fished on warm summer evenings by the sluice gates: an angler needs a ripple to hide his or her leader, otherwise the line becomes visible and scares the fish away. Quiet does this to the monofilament of stories that binds our lives. In the quiet, everything is exposed, for better or worse. My grandfather's words, because they were few, stick with me.

"I know, I'm not supposed to be smoking. It'll be our secret, Brett," he said as he took a break from dismantling the Quonset.

He was clearly out of breath. I just stared at him. Within five months of this exchange he was dead. To this day it gives me chills to think of him speaking my name. I wish I remembered the tone better. I wish I could remember more clearly what my name, spoken in his voice, sounded like, but the memory has lost its soundtrack and is mainly a scenic one now. I have a distinct memory of walking along one of the sloughs at the Cascade farm while in Montana for my grandfather's Catholic, open-casket funeral, which was attended by many—he was a popular man. The Missouri had carved the oxbow sloughs centuries earlier, and large, dying cottonwoods stood as a last testament to the river's ancient presence there. Low clouds blanketed the Big Belt Mountains and a drizzle fell over the Chestnut Valley.

A philosopher has explained of the visual nature of memory: "Memory can be considered scenic, representing a kind of imaginary landscape," which makes recalling it, in the form of story, "not only a description but rather an active interpretive redescription of an event." In other words, talking about memory is more akin to describing a film than reviewing a book. If memory is "spontaneous, represents life, and is the phenomenon of the present," then history is a "social science and a cognitive enterprise and comes with a rational reconstruction of the past." I will say this: if these flashes of memory are the stuff from which autobiography is constructed, then the medium is challenging at best, because these are really only scenic recollections, providing no sense of consistent texture or structure for me. I am not sure if they are "true," in a God's-eye sense of the word, but they are true to me. Simply, I make them true as I recall them and narrate them; they are true because I have believed them to be true for so many years. And they are true in another sense: I did not conjure them from thin air, because my parents remember them, too. My memories are more than simply *Rashomon* chaos, with each character recalling a completely different scenario: embedded in them somewhere is reality. Still, I have found that by narrating them, I have inadvertently injured them—all that remains of these memories now is the collection of versions memorialized in these pages, where they have lost so much of their visual texture.

LeRoy had dreamed for years of having a stake like the Cascade farm, a piece of land to plow, a place to live, and a place where he could hunt, his favorite passion. He told my grandmother he wanted livestock, perhaps pigs and chickens. When he died, only a flock of giant white geese evidenced this wish; my uncle Lee and aunt Sue, who inherited the farm, did not want livestock. My grandfather's life culminated with the purchase of the farm and soon after terminated. I felt pain over losing him, but I was too young for the loss to really pierce me, like it did my mother. She worshipped her father and cried for months after his death. My mother is ten years older than her closest sibling, my uncle Lee, and, as the eldest, she held the position of her father's son for years. They hunted together and farmed together. "I hated my mother, your grandmother," she once said. "I loved Dad and never left his side." But she had to now.

My grandfather had owned his first slice of farmland in Cut Bank, Montana, and my mother, as a little girl, rode horses across those windswept grasslands. This is the "almost featureless prairie" Stegner described from his youth. He observed that the Hi-Line prairie remains "notable primarily for its weather, which is violent and prolonged; its emptiness, which is almost frighteningly total; and its wind, which blows all the time in a way to stiffen your hair and rattle the eyes in your head." He continued, saying that the prairie lands of the Hi-Line and southern Saskatchewan are "quiescent, close to static; looked at for any length of time, they begin to impose their awful perfection on the observer's mind." This landscape prompted him to observe that "eternity is a peneplain." This windy eternity saturated Stegner's memories, even though those memories, the older they became, "seem uncorroborated and delusive," almost "fictitious." But what memories Stegner did believe to be real, authenticated by the sights and smells of place, are of this Hi-Line prairie. And in this same landscape, locked in my own memories of a little white-haired boy cleaning a Quonset hut alongside his dying grandfather, are the first traces of my family history of illness.

When I was in the hospital, doctors had encouraged me to think of connections between my health and my grandfather's. At forty-four, I was in fact not so much younger than he was when he became ill. A flood of disjointed visions of my grand-father's tanned leathery body haunted me at night. I vividly recalled riding in his two-tone blue Ford pickup truck on a piece of wheat-farming property we owned between Cascade and Ulm on Highway 15. The sun had turned the rolling land a hot yellow, and the buzzing and snapping of grasshoppers saturated the ripened wheat fields. Dried and cracked, the dirt holding the wheat had hardened to concrete, having received its last rain weeks or even months earlier. The pickup truck easily rolled through these fields, rocking and creaking over the dirt clumps that cluttered the primitive double track through the fields. Occasionally, my grandfather got out to crush the wheat heads in his dark calloused hands. The radio broadcast an agriculture report. "It makes chewing gum, Brett," he said as he threw it in his mouth. I relished this, and followed suit, taking the brown grains of wheat from his hand, my small fingers digging them from the dry creases in his skin, and putting them in my mouth.

One night in the hospital, a distinct memory came to me. My grandfather had just received an early-generation LED digital watch as a gift, maybe for his birthday. It was large and blocky, and the band and watch body were both made of thick black plastic, the kind that brittles in the sun. When you pressed a button on the side of the square face, the time appeared in red digits. In this particular memory, it was a bright, sunny Montana day, and I was with my grandfather, driving around the farm in his Ford. We'd stopped, and he was preparing to give himself an insulin shot because of his diabetes. Curious about the time, he looked at his watch, but it was too bright in the cab to see the LED readout. "I wonder what kind'a fool makes a watch that can't be seen in daylight," he chuckled, mainly to himself. I shook my head: what kind of fool indeed. But my eyes had zeroed in on the needle that emerged from a small cooler—I was mesmerized watching him about to poke himself the stomach. I remember this scene with almost unnerving clarity: the black plastic watch, the shining needle, the yellow-hot day, the buzzing grasshoppers, the smell of warm vinyl in the cab of the truck, the Snickers wrappers crunching underfoot on the floor, the crackle of ripened wheat.

I have since asked my mother and uncle about the watch, but they do not recall it. Neither does my grandmother, whose memory is quite good, even in her midnineties. Writing about this memory and others has forced me to scrutinize such visions carefully. Perhaps they are like the butterfly dream of Zhuangzi, a Taoist philosopher of the fourth century BCE, a dream in which reality blurs in the shifting tides of remembrance: "Once Chuang Chou dreamt he was a butterfly, a butterfly flitting and fluttering around, happy with himself and doing as he pleased. He didn't know he was Chuang Chou. Suddenly he woke up and there he was, solid and unmistakable Chuang Chou. But he didn't know if he was Chuang Chou who had dreamt he was a butterfly, or a butterfly dreaming he was Chuang Chou."

But thinking of my grandfather in the pickup that day, I remember being me, and I remember the watch. In the memory I do not switch places with my grandfather, nor do I observe him from the perspective of one of the buzzing grasshoppers. The problem is, nobody else remembers the watch. How can my recollections, then, be material for a family history of illness? Are such memories strong enough empirical evidence from which to draw medical or historical conclusions? I'd never

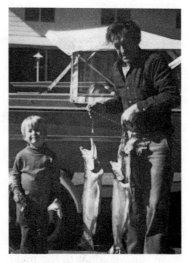

My grandfather, LeRoy Belote, and me after trout fishing, probably on Holter Lake, just north of Helena, Montana

felt as much like Zhuangzi's butterfly as when I'd been in the hospital, not sure what was real and what was not. But the memories continued to wash over me.

I remembered the death of Queen, our dutiful black lab. The dog was convulsing in the living room of our log farmhouse, scratching at the floor with her paws and then stiffening as her legs shot straight out. "Grandpa!" I screamed. He was out front, probably tinkering with a truck or some piece of farm equipment. "Dad!" my grandmother yelled, running in from the kitchen. He came into the living room in a rush and kicked Queen in the chest, hard, again and again. He got on all fours and punched the now motionless animal in her chest, trying to revive her heart. He then lowered his head and pressed his ear to her chest. I saw a tear roll down the dry wrinkles of his face, creating the illusion of a dark ravine. This rock of a man had cried. He looked at me and said nothing. I had a green John Deere toy tractor in my hand—I'd been plowing the carpet, working on my imaginary farm. I continued to do so, uncomfortably, after he left with Queen cradled in his arms. He never spoke of the dog again, even though I desperately wanted to know what he did with her dead body.

I have a handful of photographs of my grandfather, and in many he wears a silver-banded watch, not a black plastic one. But in one photograph from later years there is a black plastic watch on his wrist, though it is impossible to tell what type because of his long sleeve. I look at the photograph for historical corroboration that will substantiate my memories of the insulin incident in the pickup. I am in the picture, too, along with my young mother and my grandmother, and my grandfather is clearly not well. My mother is pouting and looks as if my grandmother has been tormenting her. My grandfather looks painfully resigned: he exudes an impatient and aloof air. I know this feeling. When I do not feel well, as I often do not, people have a tendency to annoy me, too.

Judging from scarce family pictures, I had two grandfathers around the time of my birth in 1967. One photograph, dated September 1967, is from Grandpa LeRoy and Grandma Frances's twenty-fifth wedding anniversary—the pair are jointly pushing a knife through a cake. My grandfather is stunningly handsome, the spitting image of Bing Crosby, whom, as family lore has it, he was frequently confused with in restaurants. He has a confident, radiant, shit-eating grin on his face, which his neatly cut hair accentuates. He sports a cream-colored carnation in his black jacket, and his white shirt frames an uncommonly fashionable thin maroon necktie. There is a round crystal chandelier above the couple's heads, and glass plates and a silver coffee set nearby. My mother tells me the photograph was taken in

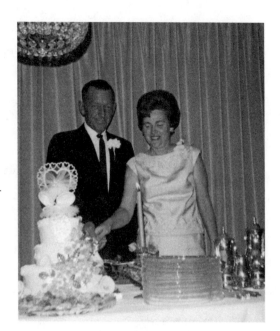

My maternal grand-
parents, LeRoy and
Frances Belote, in
September 1967 at
their twenty-fifth
wedding anniver-
sary celebration
in Great Falls,
Montana

one of the houses my grandfather built as a contractor, before
he bought the Cascade farm. My grandmother is smiling, a
little uncomfortably, as she looks at the cake; my grandfather's
eyes are screwed directly into the camera. The photograph
transports my grandfather's confidence and deserved arrogance
fifty years into the future.

Later photographs, however, from the early 1970s, depict a
different man. In these my grandfather is thin and looks tired,
with spindly legs, gaunt features, an ashen color, and slightly
sunken eyes that look away from the camera. He looks exhausted,
much older; he is always seated and always distracted, perennially lost in thought it seems to me. In none of these pictures
do his eyes pierce the camera lens, like in the September 1967
anniversary photograph. There is no confident grin; rather, he
looks annoyed and impatient.

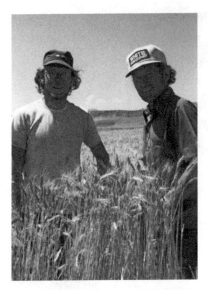

My uncle Lee (*left*) and grandfather LeRoy Belote at my family's dryland farm between Ulm and Cascade, Montana

In the later photographs from the Ulm land—the piece of farmland my family owned between Great Falls and Cascade, before buying the Cascade farm—my grandfather's hair has grown out a little, noticeable because it flares out from under his White Farm Equipment baseball cap. Gone is the military cut of his air force days. I remember this cap—I cherished opportunities to wear it. Along with my aunt Leslie, my grandfather often drove a red Massey Ferguson combine while harvesting this property, with either my brother, Aaron, or me curled up asleep in the cab. In one picture, the golden wheat is as tall as us boys, and up to the chests of my uncle Lee and my grandfather. I actually remember this photograph being taken, and I have vivid memories of my grandfather from this period. In these pictures he is thin but smiling; he had started using insulin but had not yet been diagnosed with lung cancer. He is about my current age in these photos, but the sun has significantly baked his skin. He looks far older than a man orbiting fifty years of age. Farm life can be tough on people.

— · —

Since my diagnosis with CVID, I have become even more obsessed with memory and history than is usual for a historian, and in a far more personalized way. As a historian, I constantly think about how we conceive of and narrate the past. I also think about what purposes history serves, whether for development of personal identity, questioning the status quo, or building political and societal cohesion—history, as a powerful political tool, has the unique ability to both balkanize and unify. We are nothing more than our histories, even at the visceral scale of our bodies. Shared stories are important because they

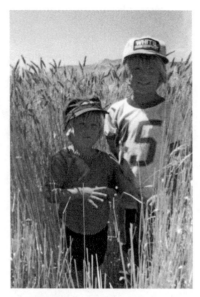

My brother Aaron (*left*) and me at my family's dryland farm between Ulm and Cascade, Montana

bind us, and the past is a far richer and more important source of such stories than the shifty present.

History has always been about empirical accuracy for me. In the end, my grandfather either wore or did not wear an early-generation digital watch, and the experiences that drift in my mind—the two of us together under the blazing sun, with grasshoppers buzzing—either happened or did not. I like to think that this is part of what Ernest Hemingway called "truth" in prose, something different than pure "description." Hemingway, when experiencing writer's block, encouraged himself with the thought that "all you had to do is write one true sentence. Write the truest sentence you know." He explained that "it was easy then because there was always one true sentence that I knew or had seen or had heard somebody say."

History is a little more complicated, because the sentences should be stylistically true, of course, not filled with "scrollwork or ornamentation," but their content should be true as well. That is, a sentence should accurately describe the empirical evidence upon which it is based. In our decrepit political age of "alternative facts" and "fake news," these distinctions are more important than ever. Today, the question of what can be known and not known through memory and history is a critically important one. Think about the fake-news moment that has become the stuff of Orwellian legend. On January 22, 2017, on *Meet the Press*, host Chuck Todd had pressed Kellyanne Conway, a senior advisor to President Donald J. Trump, about the press secretary's falsehoods regarding crowd sizes at the president's inauguration two days earlier. With her indefatigable RV-campground charm, she told Todd: "Don't be so overly dramatic about it, Chuck." She then said, "You're saying it's a falsehood, and they're giving—our press secretary, Sean Spicer, gave alternative facts to that." Unbeknownst to many at the time, Conway's comment rattled the Enlightenment rationalism that underpins our democratic society. In effect, Conway conjured a pre-Enlightenment world dominated by magic and faith and challenged the commitment that reality can be revealed and explained by empirical thinking.

With the arrival of alternative facts and their journalistic sibling, fake news, the baseline that undergirds our discourse shifted. Since then, political adversaries in the United States debate not only policy matters but also the ability to portray reality—the reliability of memory and the utility of history. It is not enough just to remember something and, therefore, believe it to be true. Historians ought to take some responsibility for teaching these basics: they need to intellectually prepare people to interrogate memory, recognize historical facts, and discern empirical reality. Most importantly, historians need to reacquaint people with how to build empirically based knowledge, and then articulate the difference between that knowledge and unsubstantiated beliefs or conspiracy theories. In a way, that is precisely what I have tried to do with this book: take the hazy ambiguity and fluid unreliability of memories, acknowledge that memories are all I've got, and then interrogate them and discipline them into a reliable and useable story—one that has medical diagnostic power or, as history, has the power to explain my world.

In the company of my students, I am old-fashioned on this matter of truth, even in the age of so-called truth-decay. If evidence demonstrates that a thing happened as you claim it did, then it's a defensible fact; if the evidence says otherwise, then, in the words of my ninety-five-year-old grandmother, it's bullshit. By our conventional definitions, if the insulin-shot episode with my grandfather happened, if he indeed had a plastic LED watch and could not read the numbers in the midday sun, then it is part of my family history of illness. But what if it never happened? "Do you have a family history of illness?" may be a routine medical question, but it is not routine for a historian who thinks about the nature of memory, history, and our ability to portray reality virtually every waking moment of his life.

— . —

Two thinkers became instrumental in how I have come to understand my own body and history, especially their ideas about how the self operates in the world. The first is twentieth-century philosopher Martin Heidegger, a brilliant man who forever tarnished his reputation by collaborating with the Nazis in Germany. Heidegger was interested in the nature of being; and for him, being was about engagement with the material world. Unlike many philosophers who focus on the transcendent cognitive abilities of human beings, Heidegger wrote of the "being-in-the-world," a person who views himself or herself solely in relationship to surrounding material realities, the people and things encountered every day. Heidegger described this relationship to the material world using two terms. The first, *thrownness*, means just that: we are thrown into our lives; we become the person we are through a particular set of material, social, economic, political, and even biological circumstances over which we have no control. In Heidegger's words, a human being "finds itself in its thrownness," which includes "finding itself in the mood that it has." In this regard, a person is "lost in its 'world'" but "not of its own accord." This is an important idea for historians because it highlights the significance of historical contextualization in crafting a narrative. In Heidegger's estimation, historical personages, the George Washingtons of the world, do not make their times, but rather their times make them.

The second of Heidegger's terms is *facticity*, which means that the "destiny" of a human being is defined by a person's relationship with "those entities which it encounters within its own world." The material world I was thrown into was filled with many good things, such as my loving parents and Montana farm life, but it was also filled with killer microorganisms in my body, environmental toxins and other pollutants, and perhaps a hereditary predisposition toward CVID. I have no control over this reality into which I have been thrown. But the "entities" with which I have formed historical relationships include more than just killer microorganisms; they also include Harvard immunologist Charles Janeway, who identified CVID in the mid-twentieth century and pioneered, at great personal cost, the lifesaving treatment. I never met him, but his historical activities are connected to my being—to my being alive, that is. The world is filled with important historical connections and convergences, ones we seldom have any control over or even discern; but such convergences are important to my family history of illness because they created the medical science, clinical practices, and therapies that allow me to survive.

The second thinker is neurophysiologist Charles Scott Sherrington. In a lesser-known chapter written in 1900 on human physiology, Sherrington discussed his interest in the relationship between consciousness and our internal organs. We tend to think of consciousness as resulting from our relationship with things and people that exist outside our bodies; we assume that the most important things we sense, such as an affectionate touch, originate from outside. But Sherrington was among the first neurologists to link consciousness to sensory experiences inside the body, building early connections between the gastrointestinal and central nervous systems. Sherrington called this nexus "the material me," a wonderfully descriptive phrase in any medical narrative. Not all sensations are "external agents," he wrote. Some are actual physical "processes of the animal body." The object of these sensations, he concluded, is "the material me." He also said that the "sensations that arise in internal organs and viscera . . . contribute a great deal" to our senses, which in turn contribute to consciousness. When we are healthy, these internal sensations are not as important as external ones in driving consciousness; but when we are ill, our internal feelings become increasingly important in how we view ourselves. This is the material me, a person built both from engagement with the world outside and from sensations emanating from within. The story of my family history of illness shifts between these internal and external worlds in order to better explain what nearly killed me.

I'll admit that I have never before embarked upon a project whose potential results I found so unnerving. In past works, the written results, or the narrative I crafted, have always been marginally interesting, perhaps useful, maybe important, but never downright terrifying. Writing this medical narrative felt like getting an important blood test done and then having to wait in the doctor's office for the results. It was with this trepidation that I began to interrogate my own past, wondering all the while what the verdict would be for my own future. When my future actually was thrown into peril, it came from a quarter I hadn't expected—even though, as I probed my health history, I realized I probably should have seen it coming.

In the summer of 2017, as I finalized this book, acrimonious political debate over health care raged in the United States, which fueled my sense of trepidation. I began to wonder, "Could my analysis of the origins of my disease be turned against me to deprive me of health insurance?" When doctors originally diagnosed me with common variable immunodeficiency in Minneapolis, President Barack Obama's Affordable Care Act was already law, and I didn't need to worry about insurance companies either discriminating against me because of a preexisting condition or placing lifetime limits on my coverage. This landmark legislation contained rights and protections ensuring that I—and others like me who fight or manage life-threatening illnesses—could not be discriminated against, that I could be insured even should I report in these pages that I inherited my disease because mutations preexisted somewhere in my genome. Unavoidably, and without my realizing it at first, this book began to intersect with political debates over health care and how we understand diseased bodies. Indeed, at its core, this book asks such questions as: "What is a preexisting illness anyway, given the complexities of genetics, epigenetics, and the chance historical circumstances of life?"

Often, disease occurs because of a series of complex convergences, ones the victim has little control over—he or she is simply *thrown* into unfortunate circumstances, to use Heidegger's word. Obviously, lifestyle choices matter, but women don't ask for breast cancer or autoimmune disease; some just get it. In this manner—as in the construction of any identity, such as gender or ethnicity or whatever—an encounter with disease, and living within a diseased body, becomes who you are and is built from interwoven biological and historical realities; some of these we have control over, others we don't. I came to think, "If people are essentially thrown into a diseased body, shouldn't illness and access to medicine be treated as a human rights issue rather than viewed as an entitlement program?" On this planet, people come in different colors, shapes, and sizes and have different languages, cultures, needs, desires, and hopes—and these factors all contribute to who we are. Illness can potentially affect all of us, and although disease is woven from biological and historical strands, there is also something physically transcendent about it, beyond the influence of our cultural milieu—which gives disease a far simpler, far more universal way to categorize people. Botanist Hope Jahren, in her memoir *Lab Girl*, explained it this way: "There are only two kinds of people in the world: the sick and the not sick. If you are not sick, shut up and help."

I remained resolved to publish this history, despite any inherent risks, if only to contribute to how we view health and disease in our lives—and this decision served as one more reminder, as if I needed one, of the importance of history.

CHAPTER 2

Immunodeficiencies

A N ABSENCE OF IMMUNOGLOBULINS, LIKE THE ONE I was diagnosed with in Minneapolis, kills people. The reason is that immunoglobulins are antibodies, and they are a vital part of a spectrum of weapons the body mobilizes to fight infection. If the body is unable to manufacture antibodies (the average immunoglobulin count for a human body is between six hundred and fifteen hundred milligrams per deciliter), relatively common bacteria, often bugs indigenous to our bodies but kept in check by our immune defenses, can cause dangerous infections, including pneumonia or sepsis. Even though antibiotics often work temporarily in such circumstances, immune-deficient bodies eventually succumb to the continual microbial onslaught. Antibodies do not comprise the entirety of our immune systems, but they are an irreplaceable part of it. Remove them and you are through.

Nobody knew the implications of tenacious bacterial infections better than Charles Alderson Janeway, whose medical career spanned from the beginning of World War II to the 1970s. Throughout his career, he was at times a bacteriologist, an infectious disease expert, and an investigatory hematologist, as well as a specialist in pediatric and family medicine. For patients with CVID, Janeway pioneered the therapeutic use of intramuscular and, later, intravenous immunoglobulin replacement therapy. That is, he sought to boost antibody levels in patients who needed them in order to combat infections. He first experimented with bovine gamma globulin, but then transitioned to human immunoglobulins after two test patients experienced what is called "serum sickness" and died. The reason why human immunoglobulins work as replacement therapy is simple: immunoglobulins derived from blood donors contain antibodies created by those good people, often thousands of good people, when they were exposed to routine bacterial and viral agents called antigens. When infused in patients like me, the antibodies of others fight infections in those patients because, essentially, they have seen the antigens before. For immune-deficient patients, it takes the cellular memory of others and an antibody village to stay alive. Janeway knew this well, and over the course of his career he constructed a medicine framework based on this basic principle.

In 1943, while Janeway was a thirty-four-year-old researcher in the lab of Edwin J. Cohn, he had a colleague, William Berenberg, inject him intravenously with gamma globulins, essentially antibodies, from some of the first human blood-fraction serums created in Cohn's Harvard lab. Cohn's lab conducted blood research for the US military, because it held enormous promise for treating wound shock, measles, and other health consequences of war. Like many important technological breakthroughs, medical or otherwise, Janeway's gamma globulin research was closely tethered to the US war effort in the

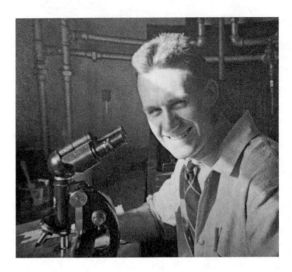

Charles Janeway behind the microscope in the bacteriology laboratory around 1938

1940s. Though not a soldier, Janeway did make sacrifices for the United States and the Allies: his injection was probably the first dose of human gamma globulins, the prototype of the "magic" medicine I received in Minneapolis, introduced into another human being. The results proved disastrous: he had a severe reaction to the serum, going into shock and developing a high fever. As Berenberg later recalled, however, this was not the last time that Janeway developed serum sickness while injecting himself with gamma globulins. Indeed, after Janeway's death in 1981, some of his colleagues hypothesized that his later struggles with what is called "hypergammaglobulinemia," when the body overproduces gamma globulins, probably resulted from this earlier overstimulation of his own immune system with repeated injections. Simply, he put his body on the front lines, and he did so mainly for children.

History can be merciless when it comes to ironies, and few could be crueler than the fact that the physician who put his life on the line to save so many other lives likely died from, at least in part, the same "magic" medicine that later became one of his most lasting contributions to medicine. However, as I began to investigate the work of Janeway, one of the people responsible for my being alive today, I realized that this instance of self-sacrifice fit squarely into his principled view of how medicine serves the global community. His story, in particular his research into what was then called "agammaglobulinemia" (today's CVID), is a part of a tangled web of events that made me who I am. I am a product of the historical events I was thrown into, including my intertwinement with Janeway's life, just as I am the product of the flesh and blood that comprises "the material me."

This is why history, as a means of knowing, can be so powerful: it has the ability, in the most complex possible sense, to discover the webs of context and connections—both those ultimately close by and those proximately far removed—that we exist within and that create who we are and define our communities. Part of my story, my historical heredity, includes war and wartime experimental medicine, blood fractionation experiments in Sweden and the United States, and cutting-edge infectious-disease medicine at Boston Children's Hospital and the Harvard Medical School. "The material me" is a product of the complex traits and predispositions passed down through my family's genetics, shared environments, and common lifestyles; but I am also a historical construction, a product of the historical network of distant actors and their web of actions that make me who I am. Just like the critical components that make up healthy blood, or the genes passed down to me by my parents, these histories are the milieu into which I was born.

— · —

While I was crawling around the cab of that red Massey Ferguson combine with my grandfather near Ulm, oblivious to the genetic time bomb ticking in my body, Janeway was living in Boston and publishing papers on "agammaglobulinemia" and experimenting with the use of immunoglobulin therapy. With the idea of historical convergences in mind, I began to investigate Janeway's gamma globulin research in the hope of understanding more about the development of my own immunological challenges. Until quite recently, people with CVID simply died: reflecting on my own family history of disease, how would I ever know who had died early of an absence of antibodies? What were the early signs or clues of the disease if the results were always the same—death—particularly before the advent of antibiotics? Before Janeway's research and clinical work, people who lacked antibodies died, and the cause of death could be any number of infections; to make matters even more complicated, many of these infections are capable of killing people with healthy immune systems, too.

The opportunity to discover answers to some of these serious questions fell into my lap. In 2015, I was appointed Edwin O. Reischauer Visiting Professor at Harvard University to teach courses in Japanese history and environmental history. Originally, I had intended to use Harvard's considerable library resources to begin a book on the history of the naval war between Japan and the United States in the South Pacific, but as I began reading additional scientific literature about CVID, I realized that its discoverer, Janeway, had been a Harvard professor. When I started to snoop around Harvard's online catalogues, I learned that Janeway's papers resided in the Countway Library of Medicine's rare books collection and the Boston Children's Hospital Archives. "What luck!" I thought. "That doesn't happen very often." With Janeway's collection nearby, I began to investigate what it was in Janeway's past, and what he saw in his young patients, that had enabled him to identify

CVID. Surely, I reasoned, Janeway's history could help me better understand my family history of illness.

If I was genetically predisposed to develop an immunological disease because of something in my family history, then Janeway was predisposed to become a doctor because of his family. His great-grandfather, grandfather, and father had all been doctors, and some of them led distinguished careers. His grandfather, for example, Edward Gamaliel Janeway, served as a medical cadet in the US Army hospital in Newark between 1862 and 1863, the height of the Civil War; afterward, he moved to New York, formally finished medical school, and performed investigatory autopsies on cadavers at Bellevue Hospital to while away the hours. In the medical community, he is remembered for describing so-called Janeway spots, or bacterial endocarditis (inflammation of the inner layer of the heart). Edward Gamaliel had one son while in New York City, Theodore Caldwell Janeway, Charles's father. Like the other Janeway men, Theodore practiced medicine in New York City. The Johns Hopkins School of Medicine appointed him professor of medicine in 1914; not long after his appointment, Theodore died of pneumonia, in 1917, at the early age of forty-five. Immediately after his father's death, Charles developed a dangerous case of appendicitis. When he recovered, there could be little doubt that his future was in medicine.

After his father's death, Charles and the Janeway family moved back to their brownstone in New York City, where Charles had been born. Young Charles had access to a privileged education, including attending high school at the Milton Academy in Massachusetts. He later recalled that the kind headmaster there, an English teacher, "took time out of his busy schedule to read aloud to me daily during a period when I was convalescing from lobar pneumonia." Charles had developed pneumonia, just as his father had, but survived the infection. He went on to attend college at Yale University, where his interests included "history, economics, social problems and the paths of philosophy and religion." His favorite Yale courses explored Johann Wolfgang von Goethe and medieval European history. Despite his passion for the humanities, in 1930 he began medical school at Cornell University—though, as we shall see, his humanities training continued to shape his medical philosophy. Two years later, he transferred to Johns Hopkins University, where he received his medical degree in 1934. Four years later, he joined the Department of Bacteriology and Immunology at Harvard Medical School. He also joined the medical staff at Peter Bent Brigham Hospital, where the distinguished Romanian medical researcher Soma Weiss mentored him.

His liberal arts education at Milton and Yale instilled in Janeway a historical view of medicine, one knit together with the moral imperative to heal a deeply unhealthy planet. In a revealing lecture tucked away in the Boston Children's Hospital Archives, titled "Looking Ahead: The Future of Medicine," a version of which was given at Brown University in 1964, Janeway explored the social responsibilities of doctors and scientific researchers and how their responsibilities dovetailed with the future of life on earth. If Janeway had been a historian, he would have been a "big" historian, because he situated history and medicine in deep geologic time. Janeway's vantage point was a cosmic one. Our species, he mused, represents a "brief manifestation of biochemical activity on an incredibly thin film of soil" covering the earth, one dependent on the energies produced by a "star of low magnitude in a huge galaxy, which itself is only a small part of an infinitely changing, expanding universe." For an audience of doctors and medical researchers, this must have been a jarring start to the lecture.

Though the earth's biofilm is thin, the sun's radiation minuscule, and the universe infinitely vast, our species, driven by our oversized brains, transforms the terrestrial world daily. This is caused in no small part by accelerating "technological change," he reasoned, to which our species must constantly adapt "if we are to save ourselves from annihilation by catastrophes of our making." Janeway labeled this predicament the "modern condition," and it shaped his views of health and the human body.

This holistic view of the modern condition, where physics, geology, biology, technology, history, and philosophy whirled together to create a violent storm of global human inequality, made Janeway a strident international activist. As I thumbed through his papers, a hodgepodge of random fragments of this man's life, I began to see a likeable medical scientist of a type nearly extinct in today's university climate, a polymath who viewed the scientific world through the lens of his earlier humanistic training. Had I lived earlier, taught at Harvard earlier, and survived pneumonia earlier, I might have found myself not only collaborating with Professor Janeway but also drinking a cold beer with him in Cambridge, after we had driven to a pub in his Volkswagen microbus—the import paperwork for which I stumbled across in his archive.

His life mission was a humanitarian one. In 1945, he worried as Cold War rhetoric between the United States and the Soviet Union ramped up. That year, when Montana senator Burton K. Wheeler and New Jersey senator Albert W. Hawkes asked US soldiers in Rome if they would like to "finish the job" in Europe by fighting the Russians, Janeway remarked, "A fine way for our elected representatives to be behaving overseas." In 1946, he wrote to President Harry S. Truman: "I am particularly concerned . . . about the problem of food for the starving people in Europe and Asia. The peace of the world will in large measure depend upon the way in which we are regarded by the rest of the world." In 1964, he wrote to President Lyndon B. Johnson, saying that the nuclear test ban treaty represented a "first step in a long struggle to lift the threat of annihilation and the tremendous economic burden of armaments from our people and all the peoples of the world." Three years later, in another letter to Johnson, Janeway criticized US foreign policy, describing it as based on the myth of a "monolithic communist conspiracy for world domination and particularly aimed at isolating and encircling China." These are big ideas for a man who spent the majority of his time looking at proteins under a microscope. Janeway built his holistic philosophy on a foundation of molecular bricks, but the edifice became grand enough to accommodate thoughts on US foreign policy, global malnutrition, and the unique challenges of the modern age. I return to Janeway's interdisciplinary views of the world's challenges in the epilogue, because they represent an important lesson of this book. A holistic perspective such as Janeway's, a combination of humanistic and scientific training, is needed more than ever if we are to have any hope of remedying our own modern condition.

This holistic view of the world influenced not only his peacenik choice in cars but also his views of the human body. Like everything about the modern condition, disease was essentially a historical artifact. Very little was "natural," strictly speaking, in Janeway's views of disease and the human body. Within this modern condition, a situation driven by technological advances on earth, there are the "have" nations and the "have-not" nations, and this basic predicament defined public health. While "have-not" nations struggle with "malnutrition and infection," he wrote, the "have" nations face the "diseases of modern society," which include "accidents, cancer, heart disease, as well as problems with emotional and social adjustment."

In some respects, improvements in living conditions and advances in medicine had caused new forms of iatrogenic bodily harm (i.e., illnesses that occur as a consequence of medical treatment), raising a series of ethical questions about the place of medicine in the modern world. "As therapeutic agents grow more powerful," he explained to his audience, having brought them from the cosmic to the clinical in his lecture "Looking Ahead," we were "beginning to see infections

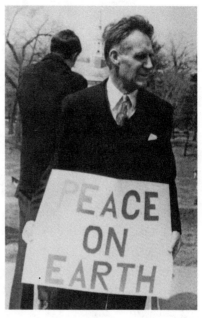

Charles Janeway protesting the Vietnam War in the Boston Commons around 1972

caused by the overgrowth of microorganisms which formerly were considered harmless normal inhabitants of the body." He continued: "When we alter the internal environment of the human body with a drug to make it inimical to the growth of [a] species of microorganism, another species or a resistant mutant of the original infecting strain may take its place." In this manner, Janeway situated the natural state of the body in the scaffolding of historical evolutionary time.

Though he repeatedly cautioned against forms of scientific reductionism—"intermolecular forces and transfer of electrons do not make a man," he explained at one point—his lecture exposes a microbiological turn in his view of the human body, a theme that influenced the direction of my family history of illness. Janeway's propensity to transcend scale would give most doctors vertigo: he was among a generation of medical scientists who viewed the body as a microbial coral reef more than as an autonomous organism. The nineteenth century had been the century of the cell, he speculated, and "microscopy was applied to the study of normal and diseased tissue"; but the "development of organic chemistry, modern protein chemistry, biochemical genetics and electron microscopy in recent years has brought us into an era of molecular biology, where processes are being analyzed in terms of the interactions of large and small molecules." As in the isolation of the gamma globulin proteins that so interested Janeway, "biological processes have been steadily dissected with finer and finer instruments down to their lowest possible terms." This is where he developed his therapeutic ideas regarding gamma globulin replacement theory: "Human health or disease in an individual requires that knowledge of how minute parts of the body work and can be manipulated by treatment must be integrated by the physician into a realistic picture of the whole man he is treating." The whole human was a being built of molecules and cells, as well as of the science, technology, philosophy, and history that shape the modern condition that so influenced the human body. Janeway's clinical analytics depended on isolating the body into its various parts, some of them microscopic, while still contextualizing it in the modern world.

Janeway took his audience on a dazzling journey through his theories on genetics, viral reproduction, and an intrusive medical science that, if placed in the wrong hands, could lead to "abuses that would even make George Orwell blanch." In the end, he anticipated the Anthropocene epoch (the current geologic epoch, in which human forces have outstripped natural forces in shaping the geophysical features of the earth), with

his thoughts on the increasing human manipulation of plane-
tary systems. With population increases sparked by new medical advances, he mused, "man will probably have to control
his environment and mold it to his purpose, but he must also
remain keenly aware of the interdependence of soil, water, and
air with microorganisms, plants and animals in sustaining the
great cycles of life on this planet." In Janeway's mind, humans
not only proved connected to the great cycles of life but also
were required to engineer them to accommodate our growing
footprint. It was with these basic humanistic, microscopic, and
cosmic assumptions that Janeway approached the study of the
body's immune system. He was a medical scientist, but one
whose humanistic training shaped his views on the body and
the role of medicine.

— . —

The science of understanding the role of antibodies in the body's
immune system started not with Janeway, however, but with the
Swedish scientist Arne Tiselius. Born in Stockholm, Tiselius
began his research career as an assistant to Theodore Svedberg
in 1925 at Uppsala University. Svedberg conducted cutting-edge
research on the molecular weight of proteins. In his lab, he
sought to discredit the idea that proteins, such as hemoglobin,
constituted a heterogeneous colloid (a solution composed of
microscopic particles) with no definite molecular weight. In
an important 1926 article, Svedberg and his colleague Robin
Fåhraeus introduced what came to be called the ultracentrifuge method, which determined the "molecular weight of
proteins based upon the measurement of sedimentation equi-
librium in a protein solution exposed to a centrifugal force."
In this method, they spun blood serum; and blood component
particles, which are not very heavy, separated one after another

according to their molecular weight. The importance of this breakthrough lies in the fact that Svedberg determined blood could be fractionated and reduced into separate components, each of which served a different purpose. As a CVID patient, I have blood and it flows plenty red, but an important component of it is missing. Svedberg's research allowed researchers to begin to see those different components, including the ones absent from my blood.

Utilizing the apparatus workshop at Uppsala University, Tiselius improved on the ultracentrifuge by introducing electrophoresis as a means to fractionate blood serum with an electrical charge. In 1930, after perfecting the method, Tiselius completed his doctoral dissertation on electrophoresis; but only six years later, after a brief foray into zeolite research at Princeton, did the Swedish scientist turn his attention once again to fractionating blood serum. To do so, Tiselius unveiled his "electrophoresis apparatus for the moving boundary method." As he later wrote, "I picked out a sample of serum from the refrigerator, dialyzed it against a buffer solution and put it into the machine. If it worked with serum, it should work with almost everything else. After about two hours I observed four distinct schlieren bands, indicating the migration of albumin and three globulin components." What emerged from those bands eventually saved my life: four distinct blood component striations that, in a separate publication one year later, Tiselius labeled in descending order of mobility: albumin (designated alb), alpha (α), beta (β), and gamma (γ) globulins, as well as a weird fifth band called the delta (δ) anomaly. He wrote, "The fastest of these components could be identified with serum albumin. The other three are found in varying amounts in all serum globulin preparations investigated. . . . They will therefore be named α, β, and γ serum-globulin." These are the protein components of human blood. The most important one for our purposes is the gamma (γ) globulin band, because that is where antibodies are located.

Subsequently, various improvements were made on the electrophoresis method and its apparatus, but the purpose was the same. One year later, Tiselius and another colleague, Elvin Kabat, highlighted the applied benefits of the separate globulin components, because the "relationship of antibodies to these components is of considerable importance." In 1938, they linked the slowest-moving serum component, the gamma globulins, with antibodies, those fierce bodily gladiators that fight microbial infections. Later, through more elaborate electrophoresis methods, researchers created even more precipitin bands out of blood serum, but gamma globulins marched to their own drummer and always moved as a homogenous band. This is because gamma globulins are a family of proteins almost exclusively composed of antibodies created when the body is exposed to an antigen. When I get an infusion of immunoglobulins at Bozeman Health Deaconess Hospital, I am receiving antibodies created by other bodies when antigens invaded them. Hopefully, the same invaders of my body once invaded other bodies, and those people graciously decided to give blood. Their antibodies stand guard over my weakened immune defenses. Tiselius, though never publicly speculating on the medical application of his discovery, did explain that many medical scientists proved interested in his research, including Edwin J. Cohn, who sent "a telegraphic order" from Harvard University. Cohn, as the reader may recall, was Janeway's mentor at Harvard during the war. That antibodies were linked to gamma globulins was of particular interest to Cohn's Harvard lab. As for Tiselius, he received a Nobel Prize in 1948 for the electrophoresis research, much as his mentor, Svedberg, had over two decades earlier for the ultracentrifuge. Fractionating blood was big-league science.

Interest in blood fractionation expanded dramatically during World War II. In 1940–41, Cohn's Harvard lab fractionated blood plasma in order to produce purified albumin, one of the components yielded by Tiselius's apparatus. Next, the National Research Council tapped Weiss, of the Peter Bent Brigham Hospital, to test some of Cohn's fractions, and Weiss placed Janeway in charge of clinical testing. In 1941, Harvard built a fractionation plant, while the laboratories of Armour and Company, the Chicago meatpacking giant and centerpiece of the Union Stockyards, designed a separate plant to produce crystalline bovine plasma. That same year, Janeway administered small doses of bovine albumin to five test subjects; one year later, researchers administered bovine albumin to some two hundred subjects from the Norfolk Prison Colony. When two men died from serum sickness, researchers abandoned the trial infusions. By March 1943, researchers had abandoned experimentation with bovine albumin altogether in order to focus on human albumin. In the battlefield, albumin, the most prominent plasma protein, effectively treated blood loss, shock, severe burns, and other common wartime wounds.

Paralleling the unsuccessful trials with bovine albumin were the trials with human albumin, and the results of the latter proved far more promising. In the spring of 1941, Janeway spearheaded the human-albumin-testing program at Peter Bent Brigham Hospital. According to a US Army official, Janeway's patient, a twenty-year-old with extensive injuries, "appeared quite groggy and irrational when I first saw him, but 12 hours later he was very clear mentally and appeared to be feeling better." With blood being spilled in the battlefields across the Pacific and Atlantic theaters, the US armed forces prioritized their interest in Harvard's albumin project. The US Navy required a "safe, stable, compact blood derivative, immediately available without reconstitution for emergency use," and Cohn's lab appeared to be the most encouraging. In fact, immediately after Pearl Harbor, dried human plasma from the Harvard lab was flown to Hawaii. Researchers delivered the human albumin to several Pearl Harbor casualties, after which they reported that "all seven patients were given albumin, and all showed prompt clinical improvement." By January 1942, National Research Council officials recommended the clinical use of albumin to the surgeons general of the army and navy.

Harvard researchers proved interested in more than just albumin, however. Using Cohn's Harvard lab serum fractions, researchers sought to make subfractions in order to create "useful and stable concentrates," as well as to harness the "many antibody molecules" in the gamma globulin fraction. These might be put to clinical use, they reasoned. The opportunity to test the clinical properties of gamma globulins came in the form of an epidemic of measles in Philadelphia in the winter and spring of 1942–43. The gamma globulins appeared to fight measles: in just under half of the thirty patients injected after the measles rash had started, the gamma globulins modified the disease; in nearly all of the patients injected when Koplik's spots (white lesions that appear before the measles rash) had already appeared, the gamma globulins modified the progress of the disease. Researchers from Cohn's Harvard lab concluded that gamma globulins with high concentrations of measles antibodies "may be of considerable therapeutic value in the early stages of measles," particularly if the gamma globulins were "obtained from pools of plasma drawn during the early stages of measles convalescence." In other words, the gamma globulins proved particularly effective when the blood pool was drawn from a population previously exposed to measles. With the results of the Philadelphia research under its belt, Cohn's Harvard lab recommended "human immune serum globulin" to the US armed forces in March 1943. But even at this early date, Cohn saw well beyond the military application of gamma globulin infusions.

As a member of the Blood Substitutes Sub-committee of the National Research Council, Cohn appreciated how university research could contribute to the US war effort. "This is the form of civilian advisory function which President Lincoln envisaged in creating the National Academy of Sciences," he wrote in 1945, "and it is to be hoped that it will be the form of the agencies which will advise Government regarding the medical sciences in the postwar world." He envisioned an interconnected knowledge-making machine, where university researchers fed results to the government, which then crafted public policy and national-security decisions based on the information. When the war had finally concluded, there would be, according to this vision, a kind of collective immunological effort, where pooled blood plasma would enhance the national immune system, particularly in controlling children's diseases. "The control of infectious diseases by passive immunization with γ-globulins may well be the largest need of a civilian population for a blood derivative," wrote Cohn, "and one to which a civilian population can be expected to contribute in the interests of the modification and control of a children's disease." With the advent of such organizations as the American Red Cross, which had collected 13.3 million pints of blood during the war, and the American Association of Blood Banks, established in 1947, the United States could create a blood pool sufficient to serve the common good through the harnessing of different blood derivatives. Each component of the blood, Cohn thought, had the potential to be a "therapeutic agent" to fight some sort of disease and ought to be used in a manner most economical and advantageous to society as a whole.

It is Cohn's vision of a national donor pool large enough to provide blood derivatives for therapeutic purposes that flows through plastic hoses and needles into my veins at the hospital. In 1942, experts considered only Armour Laboratories and Lederle Laboratories capable of producing plasma-derived proteins such as gamma globulins; but eventually the Upjohn Company, Eli Lilly Laboratories, E. R. Squibb, Cutter Laboratories, and Sharp and Dohme were contracted to produce blood derivatives in the United States. Once the war ended, however, production tapered off, in large part because, without blood spilling in the war, the market for blood derivatives, which are extremely expensive to create, did not exist. As Robert Cutter of Cutter Laboratories observed, "When you'd take the military out of it, the demand for these products among [the] civilian medical profession would not be sufficient to maintain the very expensive process of round-the-clock preparation. And getting the commercial blood . . . is a very important problem of supply, a very difficult problem." Regardless, Cutter Laboratories, founded in 1897, began plasma fractionation in 1942 and continued to produce blood derivatives until 1974, when Bayer AG purchased it. The immunoglobulin product that nurses pump into my veins is called Privigen, which is produced by CSL Behring, founded by German scientist Emil von Behring in 1904. Immediately after the war, Behring began producing plasma derivatives from blood sources in Europe for the US military. By 1949, he produced an intramuscular immunoglobulin and began the manufacture of a wide range of blood derivatives, including Privigen. Blood derivatives are indeed expensive, as my half-day hospital visit runs about ten thousand dollars; but they also prove a lifesaver for people, such as myself, with compromised immune systems.

In the 1940s, Janeway, while researching in Cohn's Harvard lab, had these gamma globulins on his mind in a very big way, particularly with respect to the promise the research held for fighting infectious disease during the war. In June 1945, he wrote to a colleague: "The plasma fractionation program has continued to expand[,] and with the general appreciation that maybe albumin is pretty good stuff and . . . that gamma globulin will prevent infectious hepatitis[,] . . . I think we can feel that we have made some contribution to the war effort." In his own studies, Janeway focused on the antibody content of gamma globulins. When the flu made its rounds through the population, for example, "it was found last winter that the titer of antibodies to influenza A rose in preparations derived from blood collected after the cessation of an epidemic due to this virus." In other words, there is a logical and local seasonality to the antibodies that gamma globulin contains. Otherwise, gamma globulins showed "considerable uniformity of antibody content despite the collection of blood at different seasons and in widely separated localities." He noted that since "the pools from which these samples are derived represent from 2,000 to 6,000 donors, the antibody levels should be fairly representative of the immunity of the group rather than a few exceptional individuals." Janeway had come to reflect Cohn's view regarding a kind of national immunology, one in which the immunological needs of the few could be bolstered by the antibodies of the many.

It was at this juncture—in 1946, immediately after Janeway accepted the position as physician-in-chief at Boston Children's Hospital—that he had Berenberg give him an intravenous infusion of gamma globulins because the intramuscular version had proved so painful for children. Janeway experienced serum sickness from the infusion, and it would be years before physicians attempted the intravenous version of gamma globulins again. It is unsurprising that, after the war, Janeway traveled to Sweden, where he met Tiselius and brought back a fractioning apparatus. With it, Janeway, together with his colleague David Gitlin, as well as Leonard Apt and Colonel Ogden Bruton, identified the disease "agammaglobulinemia" (or CVID). In 1952, they described a condition characterized by an "absence of serum gamma globulins" in children, one that caused deadly microbial infections. "We wish to present an entity," they began in dry clinical language, "not previously described, that is characterized by recurrent severe bacterial infection associated with almost complete absence of serum gamma globulins but with normal total protein concentration." They introduced readers to three boys, all about nine years old, who had had "multiple infections since infancy or early childhood." Among the boys' illnesses were serious microbial infections, "including pyoderma, purulent conjunctivitis, otitis media, purulent sinusitis, pneumonia, meningitis, acute arthritis, and sepsis—all with bacteremia," the presence of bacteria in the blood. They explained that, in all cases, the most common microorganisms in these acute infections had been all-too-familiar culprits such as *Haemophilus influenzae*, the bacteria that nearly killed me in Minneapolis. "Although the infections have been severe and the patients often critically ill," they continued, "they have usually responded promptly to antibiotic and sulfonamide therapy." I knew the rest of the story before I even finished Janeway's article: although they initially responded to antibiotic therapy, the infection being treated returned, or some other opportunistic infection took over, when the course of antibiotics was completed. Janeway and his colleagues were describing my life over the previous decade.

I feel for those boys, I really do. They appear in the first description of the disease, published in 1952. Janeway and three other authors reported that "one boy had sepsis 18 times, with eight types of pneumococci obtained on blood culture on 10 different occasions." Doctors tried sulfadiazine and polysaccharide treatments, as well as the injection of pneumococcal vaccines, but nothing controlled the infections. They scoured the boy's blood work for traces of antibodies, but none could be found. They gave him a typhoid vaccine, but noticed, to their amazement, that no typhoid antibodies synthesized, even after the shot. Then, with the Tiselius apparatus, they ran an electrophoretic analysis of the boy's blood serum, which revealed the "absence of gamma globulins." Consequently, the "boy [had] been given 3.2 gm. of human gamma globulin intramuscularly at monthly intervals, with no other prophylactic measures, for 14 months and [had] had no further attacks of sepsis." The "magic" medicine, administered by a shot, worked for this young boy, just as the intravenous form had for me. "It is postulated that these children have a congenital defect of the plasma proteins analogous to hemophilia or afibrinogenemia," they conjectured. "The entity has probably not been recognized previously because specific methods for the detection of serum gamma globulins were lacking and because severe infections contracted by such children were usually fatal prior to the era of chemotherapy."

This last statement—"because severe infections contracted by such children were usually fatal"—is what makes a family history of illness so hard to write when it comes to CVID: any relative I might have had who suffered from an absence of gamma globulins never would have been diagnosed, because blood fractionating technologies did not exist. And he or she would have died before the test could have been conducted anyway. When those University of Minnesota doctors asked me for my family history of illness, what could they have been thinking? It is more like a family history of death by bacterial infection.

In 1953, a year after the first description of the disease was published, a special correspondent for the *New York Times* reported the announcement of the "new disease" at an annual meeting of the Association of American Physicians in Atlantic City. According to the article, the disease "leaves the body of the victim without defenses against invading bacteria. Unlike normal individuals, who possess the ability to build up specific immunity against an infectious disease after a mild attack, these victims never develop this immunity." Janeway, in his announcement of the discovery, emphasized that in some respects identifying the disease was made possible by penicillin, because before the advent of the germ theory and the birth of antibiotics, victims simply died after suffering a severe infection. With penicillin, physicians had discerned that some people had the ability to fight infections after antibiotics, while others experienced recurring bouts with the disease. "Before the days of penicillin," explained Janeway in Atlantic City, "these patients must have succumbed to the extremely severe infections, which either initiated or first manifested the condition." In other words, CVID, or at least its identification, appears to fit Janeway's description of the modern condition, where medical advances, such as the birth of antibiotics, created the existence of a new disease and potential cures. Before penicillin, tons of people died from infections; after penicillin, mostly people with immunological problems did. In my family history of illness, I was searching for ancestors who had "succumbed to the extremely severe infections," so cause-of-death records would be crucial.

This is where this medical history gets frightening, because CVID, before the past couple of decades, left only death in its wake. In 1956, Gitlin and Janeway created an early profile of the disease that would one day put me in the Minneapolis hospital. "Agammaglobulinemia is a syndrome manifested by severe recurring bacterial infections in association with a marked deficiency of circulating plasma γ-globulin," they wrote. "Since almost all of the antibodies of human plasma are in the γ-globulin fraction, the occurrence of bacterial invasion is considered to be a direct consequence of the extreme paucity of this protein, and hence of antibodies, in the circulation." Importantly, in the children they had studied, "gamma globulin administered intravenously or intramuscularly to these children was catabolized or degraded at a normal or even slower than normal rate, indicating that the defect is a failure in γ-globulin synthesis." In other words, the bodies of these children were not making the gamma globulins and then somehow destroying them; rather, their bodies were simply not producing them. The problem lies in plasma cells, which both Gitlin and Janeway believed to be "intimately implicated in the production of antibodies and hence of γ-globulin." Postmortem autopsies of children who succumbed to CVID, and there were many, revealed a "complete absence of plasma cells from tissues where they are usually present—such as the lymph nodes, spleen, and the lamina propria of the intestines." The plasma cells needed to make antibodies were absent in these kids, and this killed them.

According to Gitlin and Janeway, the disease took two forms: congenital and acquired. Congenital CVID almost exclusively occurs in males, making it a "sex-linked recessive characteristic." In three of the nineteen cases that Gitlin and Janeway studied, "there was a history of other male siblings in the immediate family having succumbed to bacterial infections within the last ten years despite antibiotics." In some families, more than one male child had the disease; and in other instances, nephews and other male relatives had the disease. In its congenital form, CVID feeds on the men of a family, so tracking the disease in my family, if my form was congenital, meant investigating the men on my mother's side, such as my grandfather. Acquired CVID, on the other hand, manifests itself in adults ranging from about seventeen to seventy-one years old and occurs mainly in men, but also in some women. The acquired variety has a different symptomology. With the congenital variety, meningitis (inflammation of the protective membranes of the brain and spinal cord), septicemia (blood infection), pyoderma (bacterial skin infection), and otitis media (inflammation of the middle ear) remained painful features of the illness; with the acquired variety, gastrointestinal symptoms and pneumonia proved the most common ones. "In the past two years," Gitlin and Janeway wrote, "at least two patients of the ten described have succumbed." An 80 percent chance of living—these are not horrible odds, I guess.

In 1957, Gitlin and Janeway explored the hereditary nature of the disease, providing the path of genetic breadcrumbs that I followed as I assembled my family history of illness. While investigating the hereditary dimensions of the disorder, they discovered that, with the congenital form, "many of the families' brothers or maternal uncles of the patients had died of what appeared to be agammaglobulinemia." They continued: "It is now clear that agammaglobulinemia is a hereditary disorder." Whether the acquired form, "like diabetes, is inherited as a tendency which manifests itself only later in life," perhaps triggered by environmental causes or even stress, remained unclear. In other words, there is a critical distinction between the congenital and acquired forms of the disease, which would alter my approach to the historical investigation of my ancestors. The congenital form was hereditary, plain and simple; the acquired form included a hereditary propensity for the disease, but required something environmental to trigger it. Perhaps it was a lot like diabetes, an ailment that had plagued my grandfather until his death.

My first order of business was to determine whether I had traces of CVID as a child, and this would involve interrogating my memory and childhood medical records. Did I exhibit symptoms as a young child? Did any medical records survive from my past? If not, then when did the symptoms start? These three questions drove me to probe my memories and documents related to my past in order to retrieve visions I had not thought about in years. This is an important exercise, because memory is the foundation of history. Even in firsthand accounts of historical incidents, some remembering is involved; and I needed to understand how memory works, because mine felt so spotty. Can memories be relied upon when drafting a family history of illness, one with real clinical implications? These and a host of other questions were my guides as I tried to remember when I first felt the onset of CVID.

CHAPTER 3

Modalities

M Y EARLIEST THREE MEMORIES ARE ONLY FLASHES. They are brief visual projections in my mind, with only patchy audio portions and no distinct chronological waypoints. I have no control over when they come and go; they have a life of their own. I know their likely order only because I know we lived in a string of West Coast cities stretching from Seattle to San Francisco after we left Bozeman. I believe my earliest distinct memory is from Seattle, where we moved immediately after my father graduated from college. We had an old Tudor- style brick home with a lovely gabled roof, located close the Highway 520 overpass in the Montlake area, near the Lake Union canal and across from the university.

I have a distinct vision of gazing upward and seeing a colos- sal overpass, a ribbon of cement nearly eclipsing the sky, with only stripes of blue shining on either side. My brother, Aaron, was born in Seattle, and my mother says that we lived there until his first birthday, so this memory is probably from my third or fourth year. I am pretty sure it is my earliest formed memory, though I also know that I have other fragments of images, disharmonized "tonalities," to use Vladimir Nabokov's term, floating in my consciousness, ones that I simply cannot place in the structured currents of time. Try as I might, I cannot recall much more than flashes of the ribbon of cement, the stripes of blue, the Lake Union canal, and the quaint Tudor home; though, within the memory of the Tudor home, I have some cloudy recollections of playing with an African American boy in a house with hardwood floors. My mother informs me that he was my best friend while we lived in Seattle, a neighborhood boy who also lived near the ribbon of cement. But these recollections are fragile, and if I try too hard to retrieve them they retreat, as a slippery apple does from a child's bobbing mouth.

In Seattle, my parents baptized me into a life spent outdoors. In one family story, my parents, after consulting their first-edition *Mountaineering: Freedom of the Hills*, planned to climb to Lake Serene at the base of Mount Index, a formidable Cascade peak close to Seattle. They fought their way up the steep trail for hours, me on my mother's back, and a heavy aluminum-framed rucksack on my father's. Then, because it was getting dark and they had not prepared to spend the night, they decided to kick out the center of a rotten log for shelter. The next day, after a cold night, my parents admitted defeat, returned to the car, and drove to Glacier Peak Wilderness, where they hiked in eight miles only to discover that they had left my baby formula on the hood of the blue Volvo. My father hiked back to the car, leaving my mother and infant me on a sheet of clear plastic in the woods. Years later he would explain to me that when he finally returned, "there you were, eating bugs, wood chips, and dirt" while my mother looked on. He mixed the formula

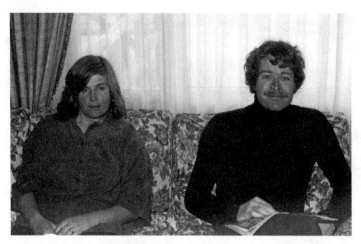

My parents, Linda and Nelson Walker

in creek water near the trail, without first purifying the water or boiling it, and I contently nourished myself in the cradle of the Cascades. I spent much of my childhood and adolescence in these mountains.

In my second early memory, I am at an alpine ski race, probably at Squaw Valley. Westinghouse had relocated my engineer father from Seattle to San Francisco in 1971, and we lived in Mill Valley at the base of Mount Tamalpais. I remember well my friend Mark and his younger sister, Yvonne, who lived in the neighborhood. Mark and I spent endless days at Stinson Beach and Point Reyes National Seashore, two blond boys running wild with only sagging white underpants loosely wrapped around our beanpole frames. The two of us were almost swept away once by a strong undertow at Stinson Beach, but my father swam into the powerful current and saved us. I learned to ride a bike here, and remember the splendid dark-purple single-speed I had for years. I have a faint image of my father pushing the back of the bike seat and then letting go. I also raced on a local swim team, where I

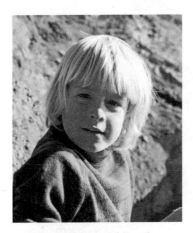

I spent most of my childhood outdoors. This picture was probably taken in the Sierra Nevada, California.

won a blue ribbon in the butterfly. While in California, we spent our winter weekends at Squaw Valley and our summer ones at Yosemite, camping and watching my father rock climb.

At Squaw Valley, I saw the five Olympic rings falling beneath us as we rode a gondola into the alpine world. "Go between the gates," my father had explained at the top of the course. I can almost feel the texture of his arm around my shoulders, his thick wool sweater scratching my bare neck. The sweater was dark gray with white snowflake designs across the chest. I did go between the gates, just as he said, and I got to the bottom first—but it was a dual slalom, and I had skied between the two courses rather than properly down one of them. What I remember next is the feeling of disappointment at being told I had not actually won the race, because I was pretty sure I had. I can also recall the texture of the cloth race bib, and how proud I was wearing it. I was around four or five years old when I started ski racing, and I continued to race even after college, when I lived in Switzerland.

My third early memory is of waking up one Easter morning in a small tent with the rest of my family. There was snow on the ground around the tent, with some yellow alpine flowers poking through; my brother and I leapt out at sunrise and scrambled through the cold white blanket, periodically blowing into our hands to warm them, looking for Easter eggs. I recall my yellow Easter basket, and the fishing pole and reel nearby, as well

as some tackle, that sparked a lifelong love affair with fishing. The
strongest part of this memory is the
bright snow and the white tree bark
from the woods, likely an aspen
grove, where we camped in Yosemite Valley. I think these are my earliest memories. I have carried these
memories with me for as long as
I can remember. They are neurological keepsakes that I have tried
to squeeze into words for the purposes of this book, but I see now
that they fit like cumulonimbus
clouds shoved into ice-cube trays.

As I began recalling my childhood, specifically my health as
a child, in order to tell my family history of illness, I forced into
words for the first time these and

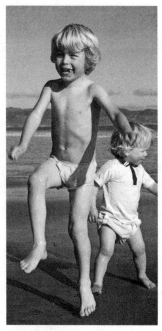

My brother Aaron (*right*) and
me during our white underpants
days in Mill Valley, California

other early, recalcitrant scenes of memory. Were other people's
first memories like mine: only visual flashes? Were other people
better able to remember? Nabokov began his memoir with the
awakening of consciousness. "In probing my childhood (which
is the next best thing to probing one's eternity) I see the awakening of consciousness as a series of spaced flashes, with the intervals between them gradually diminishing until bright blocks of
perception are formed, affording memory a slippery hold." He
speculated that the dawning of individual consciousness began
with an awareness of a "sense of time," a principal theme in
Nabokov's recounting of his life. Certainly, this sense of time is
critical to the historian's craft.

Intersecting currents of consciousness represent time for Nabokov, and history, the disciplined narration of that consciousness, the ultimate creator of self-awareness. Simply, I am history in the context of what I remember, but I am also history in the context of Janeway's immunological research and clinical solutions to CVID: the confluences of history and body intersect in such currents of time, and we can never transcend them, despite the promise of modern bourgeois autonomy from the natural world. These scenic flashes of memory originate in proteins in the brain, just as the immunoglobulins that flow through my veins are proteins. Upon recalling his earliest memory, Nabokov wrote, "I felt myself plunged abruptly into a radiant and mobile medium that was none other than the pure element of time." At this moment in his life, he came to inhabit "time's common flow," and he was rushed away by history's ceaseless current. But it was time's flow, not space's unifying plane, that defined a sense of personal identity for Nabokov: memories suspended in time, along with their more disciplined sibling, history, are the means by which we carve ourselves out from the clay-brick past that is everything else. There is truth here: for Nabokov, the Bolshevik takeover of Russia in 1917 represented truth in his life and served as the chronological waypoint for his entire story.

Nabokov lived in a world where memory and history reigned supreme. "The act of vividly recalling a patch of the past is something that I seem to have been performing with the utmost zest all my life," he recalled. And given the texture of his memoir, he proved quite skilled at the craft. I adore his ways of describing memory, as well as his way of telling family stories. "Over the shoulder of my past" is one turn of phrase, positioning memory as a dawdling companion in life, somebody with whom you might walk your dog. "One is always at home with one's past" is another acknowledgement of our inseparable connection with personal story. But there is artistry to this invention of a past. "There is, it would seem, in the dimensional scale of the world a kind of delicate meeting place between imagination and knowledge, a point, arrived at by diminishing large things and enlarging small ones, that is intrinsically artistic," he mused. Memory is the organizer of tonalities, and history is the discipliner of memory: "I witness with pleasure the supreme achievement of memory," he wrote, "which is the masterly use it makes of innate harmonies when gathering to its fold the suspending and wandering tonalities of the past." We can only hope that these memories "survive captivity in the zoo of words," Nabokov cautioned, because it is only when memory is captive in the zoo cages of words that history can be crafted and, ultimately, exhibited to oneself and the world.

I have learned that my memories do not survive captivity well. The more I sought to capture them in cages, the more they eluded me, their ever-hopeful keeper. I remember being a healthy child, never participating in any kind of sport, from skiing and swimming to cycling and sailing, that I did not pursue competitively and reasonably well, with the encouragement of my parents. In relation to my family history of illness, I remember being sick at various times, staying home from school with strep throat, for example. I was plagued often by the bacteria *Streptococcal pharyngitis* as a child. I remember being in the Mill Valley house, lying down in my bunk bed, a cool washcloth over my forehead, listening to *Magical Mystery Tour* on vinyl; and I can still taste the sweet flavor of a breaking fever, a thick film of cough syrup in my mouth, as my body's thermostat began to return to normal—today, the colorful album cover, the costumed "fab four," and my childhood fever have all merged into one psychedelic but reassuring remembrance of illness.

I remember that, at one time, my body did fight infections, because I did get well without the aid of other people's antibodies. I recall getting strep throat about once a year, often accompanied by an ear infection. I know this not because I remember the diagnosis, but because I can see the tongue suppresser, the bright headlamp, and the white-jacketed doctor taking throat cultures with his cotton swab. "We'll send these to the lab," he would casually explain to my mother. I recall the procedure of having my temperature taken by my mother before going to the doctor; when I was younger this involved a thermometer in the rear. But this did not happen all the time, and susceptibility to strep throat ran in my family. When my father first brought his college girlfriend, my future mother, to Casper, Wyoming, to meet his parents, who had recently divorced but hid the fact from him, he was hospitalized for days with it. "It was awful. I had to spend all that time alone with his divorced parents," my mother remembered. As far as I can see, I had an immunologically normal childhood, though to my knowledge I never had my immunoglobulins tested.

— · —

In 2015, my mother went through a divorce with her second husband. In the process, she began culling storage boxes from her house because she planned to relocate to a smaller house. Early that summer, she traveled to Bozeman to stay with my wife, LaTrelle, and me and brought with her a small box. "I don't know if you're interested in this or not, Brett," she said. "It's old stuff I've saved over the years, mainly from your childhood." The box was filled with old school photographs and art projects. One crude drawing of a knight on horseback was titled, in crayon, "For Dad, Love Brett." There were some spelling and grammar exercises, too, from grade school. And the box contained a surprising number of report cards and letters from teachers, most of which voiced concern about my awful performance in the classroom. But in the box I also discovered a baby-blue booklet with my name handwritten on it. This was an important find, and it promised to provide the first documentary evidence of my health as an infant.

The booklet, titled *Your Baby's Health Book*, is a prime example of the medical goodies that Mead Johnson and Company used in order to peddle its Dextri-Maltose formula to young parents. Mead Johnson introduced this product in 1912 and quickly began advertising it at American Medical Association meetings and in prominent journals, essentially turning an infant's empty stomach into a quantifiable medical condition that needed supervision. This type of booklet, which contained useful information on preparing formula and sterilizing bottles, along with a handy feeding schedule, was a classic part of their advertising campaign, because Dextri-Maltose, unlike other baby formulas, was available only through physicians. In Seattle, where my booklet originated, my physicians were Drs. Basil J. Gregores and Neil P. Duncanson, who practiced medicine on Ambaum Boulevard. By making the formula available through physicians, Mead Johnson encouraged mothers, such as my twenty-one-year-old mother, to make doctor's appointments to feed their babies. As Mead Johnson boasted to their physician clients, this "added to their practices and put money in their pockets," which it no doubt did. The booklet's front cover explains, "When visiting the doctor always take this book," which my young mother diligently did, because it contains medical jottings from my early years in Seattle, the site of my first flash of memory. If I had the congenital version of

CVID, like the young boys Janeway treated at Boston Children's Hospital, then surely there would be some signifier of my collapsing immune system in this baby-blue booklet.

If anything, at eight and a half months I was on the large size, twenty-nine inches long and a fleshy twenty-three pounds, like a smallish Chinook salmon. The results of my physical at this early date: "Exam—OK," as somebody had scribbled in the booklet. At just over fourteen months, in May 1968, I had gained two pounds and grown more than three inches; my physical results were: "Exam—Neg." Under special instructions, somebody wrote, "Accidents!, Blood Count, TB—Test, measles vaccine." The doctor reminded my mother of the eighteen-month booster and to bring me back at twenty-two months. But the remainder of the baby-blue booklet is empty, except for the immunization records section, which lists my immunizations as diphtheria, tetanus, whooping cough, poliomyelitis, smallpox, and measles, in addition to a tuberculin test, all administered in 1967. There is also an undated prescription slip in the booklet, signed by Dr. Duncanson, for ipecac syrup, to "induce vomiting," he wrote. Ipecac syrup used to be a common fixture in American homes with children, because parents used it to induce vomiting if a child accidentally swallowed a household poison. My mother told me that the syrup was prophylactic. "I was just waiting for one of you to down a bottle of Drano!" Thankfully, neither of us ever did.

"My doctor told me you didn't need breast milk. Both you and your brother were eight pounders! Your father was very social in those days, and I didn't want to be locked up in the bedroom breastfeeding you while our friends were around. In those days, mothers didn't breastfeed babies in front of people." There is a long history of women, such as my mother, exploring ways to remove their infants' mouths from their breasts.

Initially, European cultural demands for shapely breasts drove this desire; but later, increasing social mobility, the necessity of industrial labor, the availability of new feeding technologies, and pediatric debates over infant nutrition freed women from this quintessential motherly task. Over time, the simple frustration that "I didn't want to be locked up in a bedroom," that breastfeeding was burdensome and unfashionable, led women to experiments ranging from wet-nursing to the use of bottles of all shapes, sizes, and materials, at least among the moderately well heeled. Wet-nursing served as the earliest alternative to a mother breastfeeding her infant, and people around the world practiced it. But the practice has always had its detractors. Early on, one sixteenth-century Italian observer worried that the baby might "savor of the nature of the person by whom they are suckled," rather than the nature of the mother. By the eighteenth century, this line of reasoning became a powerful argument against wet-nursing.

It turns out that the Western female breast has a long, complex history. As historian Londa Schiebinger has observed, the "female breast evoked deep, wide-ranging, and often contradictory currents of meaning in Western cultures," and some of those currents ran straight through my mother's decision to not breastfeed me. Both before and after Carl Linnaeus identified the female breast as the essential marker of the class Mammalia in 1758—"Mammalia, these and no other animals have *mammae*," he wrote—Europeans extolled the cultural symbolism, as well as the moral and medical benefits, of women's breasts and the milk they provide. By the early eighteenth century, the fully developed female breast had emerged as a symbol of *Homo sapiens*, and many came to believe that children acquired important individual traits from breast milk. Linnaeus, the father of Western taxonomy, believed that certain heroic figures became

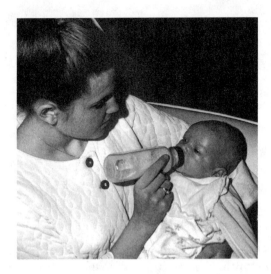

My mother, Linda,
bottle-feeding me in
Bozeman, Montana

courageous when they suckled bravery-laced breast milk from
a lioness, for example. Consequently, many important figures
became vocal opponents of wet-nursing, which had become
widespread by the eighteenth-century. By the 1780s, affluent
mothers in Paris and Lyon were sending upward of 90 percent
of their children to the countryside to be breastfed by peas-
ants, whom the wealthy viewed as closer to nature and, hence,
healthier. Sending nursing children to the countryside might
have freed up valuable time for these women, but it also led
to heightened rates of infant mortality. As European countries
from Denmark to France became concerned about declining
populations, the practice of wet-nursing fell squarely into the
crosshairs of state sanctions and medical pronouncements.

In 1752, while watching his own children nurse at their
mother's breast, Linnaeus, a physician by training, had come to
believe that wet-nursing violated the "laws of nature." He also
cautioned that most wet nurses came from the impoverished
and filthy countryside, where horrible diseases and inadequate

nutrition translated into poor-quality breast milk. But gender politics also proved a powerful driver in the campaign against wet nurses: it was in the eighteenth century that gynecologists and obstetricians, usually men, slowly replaced midwives, always women, and these men attached new, and highly gendered, significance to breastfeeding. These new professional physicians allied themselves with cultural forces that advocated breastfeeding; and by the late eighteenth century, physicians in France and Germany supported laws that forced healthy women to breastfeed. In 1793, the French National Convention decreed that only mothers who nursed their children were eligible for state aid. But an additional reason why wet-nursing fell out of fashion in Europe was that animal milk and baby formula had become safe alternatives to sending children to the countryside to feed. And at this juncture, we take one step closer to understanding my mother's decision to not breastfeed me. My young parents may have thought they had autonomously decided to feed me Dextri-Maltose, based on what was buzzing in pediatrics, but they had been thrown into a centuries-old historical debate over feeding infants that was then trending in favor of baby formula.

Of course, using animal milk to feed infants is an ancient practice. Earthen vessels with nipplelike spouts, retrieved from ancient infant graves, have revealed traces of animal milk after chemical analysis. Early Europeans used perforated bull's horns to feed infants milk, while the eighteenth century witnessed devices crafted from silver and pewter. In 1770, a physician at the Middlesex Hospital in London designed the "bubby pot," which delivered milk to babies with the aid of sponge or rag nipple. In 1851, the first glass bottle, with a cork nipple, was developed in France. Shortly thereafter, natural rubber nipples, basically polyisoprene elastomers, replaced cork ones.

Milk from a variety of animals most commonly made its way into infant guts through such devices, a process aided by the development of evaporated milk in 1835. Two decades later, Eagle Brand condensed milk appeared on market shelves, and it became a popular infant food. In 1865, a German chemist developed and marketed a synthetic alternative composed of cow's milk, wheat and malt flour, and potassium bicarbonate, and within two decades nearly thirty brands of infant food became available in liquid and powdered forms in many parts of the world. In 1891, Walker-Gordon Farms in New Jersey began the production of "clean milk," or cow's milk that more closely resembled human milk, made under the most hygienic circumstances possible. But even with such devices and procedures, artificial nipples proved breeding grounds for dangerous bacteria; some estimate that in the nineteenth century, one in three artificially fed infants died within the first year of life. Infants have fragile immune systems, and they would have been no match for big-league bacteria. The summer months were particularly dangerous, as such bacteria bloomed in the warm temperatures. At roughly the same time, however, scientists Louis Pasteur and Robert Koch began hypothesizing about the role of microorganisms in causing deadly infections and mortality, and the germ theory of disease gradually replaced humoral "miasmic theories" in explaining the etiologies of human morbidity and mortality.

Subsequently, by 1912, easy-to-clean rubber nipples became widely available, and the invention of the kitchen icebox allowed mothers to safely store milk. By the 1940s and 1950s, vitamin-fortified, milkless varieties of infant formula were commonly obtainable, which led to a dramatic decline in breast-feeding, particularly in Europe and the United States. The statistics are incomplete, but in the 1930s, American mothers breastfed approximately 70 percent of firstborn infants; and in the 1940s and 1950s, the number decreased to around 50 percent. In the late 1960s and early 1970s, when I was born, mothers breastfed only 25 percent of infants within the first week, and 14 percent after the second and third months of life. The overwhelming bulk of the formula was commercially produced rather than homemade. It was into this historical moment that I was thrown, the high-water mark of the United States' use of commercially manufactured formula. The use of infant formula has always proved a double-edged sword for a variety of reasons, and even those reasons have changed over time. The one I want to explore here is the role of breast milk in immunological modulation.

Like their eighteenth-century counterparts, doctors now recommend breastfeeding babies. In the past four decades, physicians have identified obesity, atopic syndrome (hyperallergic conditions), and diabetes as some of the possible health consequences of formula feeding. But the most alarming consequence is immunological, which naturally drew my attention to formula use in my family. Could the popularity of baby formula in the 1960s be part of my family history of illness? Did my parents' use of baby formula somehow contribute to my later development of CVID? To answer this question, we need to briefly review how the body's immune system works. Importantly, when Charles Janeway viewed the body's immune system under a microscope, what he saw was a highly complex world, one that involved microbiological alliances between varieties of organisms that call the body home.

— · —

The immune system can be divided into two broad spheres: the innate and the adaptive. The innate immune system rapidly

responds to protect the body from bad microorganisms by utilizing mucosal and epithelial (tissue that lines the surfaces of
internal organs) walls, as well as the air, fluids, and mucus that
line these critical barriers. The microorganisms in our guts and
respiratory tract also contribute to our innate immune system,
through a Darwinian drama of probiotic competition: in the
law of the gastrointestinal jungle, good flora tries to outcompete
bad flora for floor space in the gut. In a well-developed gut, one
inhabited by healthy probiotic flora, there is not much room for
bad flora to spread. And to stop those that do, phagocyte cells
patrol this bodily jungle, acting as sentinels and engulfing bad
microorganisms within tissue and along mucosal barriers.

The adaptive immune system functions in concert with the
innate immune system, though it develops more slowly over
time and with exposure to diverse antigens. Consequently,
infants have underdeveloped adaptive immune systems. In the
adaptive immune system, phagocyte cells are nonetheless present, mobilizing effector cells, including effector B-cells, which
are a kind of plasma cell or white blood cell and which secrete
antibodies, the ones that my body has stopped manufacturing.
These B-cells are critical to the immune system because they
are memory cells: they have the ability to remember disease
agents and prevent future infections. Colonel Ogden Bruton—
who together with Charles Janeway, David Gitlin, and Leonard
Apt had published a paper about agammaglobulinemia (today's
CVID) in 1952—discovered an affiliated primary immunodeficiency disease later called Bruton's syndrome or X-linked
agammaglobulinemia, which involves these B-cells.

Bruton's syndrome occurs when the process of white blood
cell formation fails to include mature B-cells. Bruton, chief
of pediatrics at Walter Reed Army Hospital, had admitted an
eight-year-old boy who suffered from repeated severe infections,

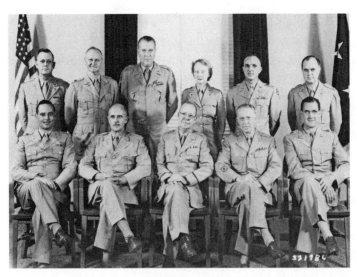

Ogden Carr Bruton was chief of pediatrics at Walter Reed Army Hospital. He is standing far right in this July 1948 photograph. Bruton was involved with Charles Janeway in the discovery of agammaglobulinemia (today's CVID), and he discovered Bruton's syndrome.

including pneumococci sepsis, pneumonia, upper respiratory problems, gastrointestinal upset, inner ear infections, and severe joint pain. Penicillin and sulfonamide treatment led to temporary improvement, but then the infections and high fever returned. When Bruton discovered an absence of gamma globulins, he administered intramuscular human serum globulin. Subsequently Bruton observed, "For the past 14 months the patient has had monthly injections of gamma globulin, without benefit of other prophylactic measures, and has suffered no attack of sepsis." In 1993, researchers linked Bruton's syndrome to a mutation of the Bruton's tyrosine kinase gene, which blocks B-cell development. Because this syndrome occurs as a result of an X-chromosome mutation, the disease is more common in little boys, such as Bruton's eight-year-old patient, because all men possess one X-chromosome, whereas only some homo-zygous women do. Given the importance of Bruton's tyrosine kinase to the immune system, it is hardly surprising that it has become the target of new treatments for B-cell malignan-cies, such as chronic lymphocytic leukemia and mantle cell lymphoma.

It turns out that memory is important at multiple bodily lev-els, because B-cells tell stories. B-cells, when they have devel-oped properly, remember past infections and secrete antibodies, just as historians research past human experiences and secrete narratives of them. Infants with congenital Bruton's syndrome or CVID develop virtually no adaptive immune system, because memory cells and antibodies are not created in response to pathogens. Every time bacteria invade and infect them, their white blood cells secrete no antibodies and never remember the experience. In all, the human immune system is pretty serious business and must be able to aggressively defend itself without accidentally turning on its cellular self; "turning on its cellular self" is the basic definition of autoimmune disorders.

Within the innate and adaptive portions of the immune sys-tem, there are three main activities. First, the phagocyte and natural killer cells, and their arsenal of cytokine and interferon signalers, are released to fight dangerous bacteria. The second activity is the humoral response of B-cells, plasma cells, and their immunoglobulin secretions. The third is the response of the flora in our guts and respiratory tract. All these innate and adaptive branches fight in a coordinated effort to protect the body from bacteria and viruses, which constantly try to get a foothold in our bodies. As the final lines of the 2005 movie ver-sion of H. G. Wells's classic *War of the Worlds* explain about the demise of the Martian invaders: "They were undone, destroyed, after all of man's weapons and devices had failed, by the tiniest creatures that God in his wisdom put upon this earth. By the toll of a billion deaths, man had earned his immunity, his right to survive among this planet's infinite organisms." It is a trenchant observation, but a terrifying one for those of us who have lost that right.

In the case of bacterial invasion, such as that of the *Haemophilus influenzae* that spread in my body and ultimately caused the pneumonia and pleural effusion that nearly killed me, immunological first responders include small cationic proteins called defensins, white blood cells called leukocytes, and ever-present antibodies, each of which plays a role in fighting infection. These cells sense trouble and travel from the blood to the site of initial bacterial infection to establish an immunological beachhead, usually on mucosal and epithelial walls. Phagocyte cells such as neutrophils and monocytes, both of which are produced in the bone marrow, are able to sense bacteriological infection in the body and migrate to the site to fight the invading microorganism. Along with immunoglobulins, phagocyte cells also fight more systemically invasive bacteria, in addition to localized troublemakers, but all these systems work together in a properly functioning immune system.

As you may have noticed, immunoglobulins are critical to defending the body from infection, and newborns produce precious few of them, particularly gamma globulins, the ones so painstakingly studied by Janeway. Memory T-cells that have been exposed to antigens, and which remember them, are important for fighting reoccurring infections, but infants do not generate them. This deficiency is partly overcome symbiotically by the mother's immune system, via immunological transference through the placenta and through mother's milk. This creates a passive immunity to infections, much like my monthly infusions do. Gamma globulins develop slowly in infants, and by the time children are a year old their gamma globulin levels are about 60 percent of adult levels. Not until about age five does a child develop the immunoglobulin repertoire of an adult, after his or her adaptive immune system matures through incremental exposure to various microorganisms, the endemic disease pool of a community. At an individual level, only after about age five has the child, as *War of the Worlds* puts it, "earned his immunity, his right to survive among this planet's infinite organisms."

Breast milk is important for boosting an infant's underdeveloped immune system in numerous ways, something pediatricians began observing as early as the turn of the century. Ernest Moro was one such pediatrician. In 1903, he was the first to identify the important immunological qualities of breast milk. Born in Ljubljana, Slovenia, he was among the earliest medical researchers to discover that breastfed children have stronger antibacterial capabilities in their blood than bottle-fed ones do. When he emerged on the scene in Europe, pediatrics, as a medical field, had only recently separated from internal medicine. Theodore Escherich, Moro's teacher, held the first chair in pediatrics in Graz, Austria, and he quickly became a global leader in children's medicine. Escherich had focused on infant intestinal bacteria and the physiology of digestion, and Moro dutifully followed in his mentor's footsteps. In 1898, Moro determined that human milk contained digestive enzymes not found in cow's milk. In 1900, he identified the microorganism *Lactobacillus acidophilus*, which calls the human mouth and digestive track home and often exhibits probiotic characteristics (i.e., those of healthy bacteria and yeasts). Three years later, Moro opened a private children's hospital in Vienna and, working with his colleague Arthur Schlossman, a German pediatrician, discovered useful proteins, including antibodies, in human milk. By 1911, Moro became head of Children's Hospital in Heidelberg, where he served until the rise of the Nazis cut short his career. But other pediatricians followed his lead.

More recently, in the 1970s and early 1980s, medical researchers explored the role of antibodies and immunological cells in modulating an infant's nascent immune system. Niels Kaj Jerne, for example, a Dutch scientist, hypothesized in his "network theory" that only when antigens disturb the balance between specific and nonspecific antibodies is an immune response launched in the body. With medical researchers focusing on immunological and probiotic effects of breast milk, it is not surprising that formula use, after reaching its high-water mark around the time of my birth in 1967, began to decline as medical information about this subject was communicated to the public. By this time, I was already gnawing on bugs and bark in the Cascades, strengthening my immune system in other ways.

Human breast milk contains a host of ingredients that assist in infant development, such as a variety of enzymes and proteins, as well as cytokines and chemokines (signaling proteins secreted by cells), which bolster the immune system, and defensins, which fight pathogenic microorganisms. Breast milk also contains hormones, such as prolactin, which assist gut development and immunological modulation. Other beneficial ingredients in breast milk include carbohydrates, antioxidants, lipids, nucleic acids, and anaerobic bacteria such as bifidobacteria, which inhabit the human mouth, vagina, and colon and serve beneficial probiotic purposes. Heavy-hitting cells such as neutrophils and macrophages, not to mention white blood cells, such as T-cells and B-cells, are also transmitted to the infant through breast milk, some of them remembering previous infections in the mother's body and carrying that memory to the infant's body to defend it.

In this respect, white blood cells, specifically lymphocytes, and antibodies in breast milk represent the adaptive immunological responses of the mother's body and, therefore, are products of the immunological experiences of the mother during her life. Though the modulating ability of lymphocytes and antibodies is limited to a brief period immediately after birth, their imprint on a person's immune system is lifelong and even dominates many genetic immunological predispositions. In this way, the immunological characteristics passed through breast milk represent an example of epigenetic evolution — that is, nongenetic characteristics acquired during the mother's lifetime that are passed to offspring. The best examples of this epigenetic predisposition are lymphocytic B-cells, some of which live for over a year and which have somatically mutated (or have gained memories) in the mother's body over the course of their lifetimes in response to environmental microorganisms. Lymphocytic B-cells produce specific adaptive immunoglobulin phenotypes such as alpha and gamma globulins, molecules bearing information about the microbiological environment, which the mother transfers to the infant. In sum, the ability of infants to combat infections depends almost entirely on the mother's immunological experiences and nongenetic inheritance, which give the offspring an evolutionary advantage. Presumably, a baby lives in the company of many of the same infectious bugs as his or her mother and so survives.

My mother's immunological experiences are part of my family history of illness, because the lymphocytic B-cells and antibodies I inherited from her represented specific phenotypes born from her body's exposure to microorganisms. My mother transferred antibodies to me through her placenta, but I was deprived of the numerous immunological benefits of breast milk, as were millions of other infants born around the world.

Instead, I was fattened on the larder of Mead Johnson. But I have concluded that a lack of breast milk did not cause the CVID that nearly killed me in Minneapolis over four decades later. If this lack were capable of causing CVID, the latter would be far more common, and I would have acquired it earlier. Regardless, elements of my innate and adaptive immune systems are products of epigenetic, not just genetic, inheritance, and this has complicated how I must approach the writing of my family history of illness, a topic I return to in the epilogue. Family experiences, such as my shared immunological history with my mother, are just as important as genetic explanations or evidence of the disease in my extended family. But this was the immunological development of "the material me" when I was thrown into the world, a product of family genetics, experiential epigenetic inheritances, and historical circumstances such as baby-feeding trends and pediatric medicine in the twentieth century, trends my parents and I found ourselves completely swept up in as I entered this world.

— . —

By the time we moved to the Bay Area in 1971, I was off of formula; but was there any evidence that baby formula had affected my immunological development? Did a teacher observe that I was sickly at age four or five, when my immune system was finally growing legs of its own? Again the box of family trinkets and documents my mother gave me proved informative. In December 1973, when I was six years old, one of my first-grade teachers at Marin Terrace School in Mill Valley penned the earliest surviving trace of the young me, a hieroglyph in the bone cave of my cognitive life. She observed, as she probably did with all her students, that I was in "constant motion" and did well in class after I "settle[d] down and concentrate[d] on the task at hand."

I flew through the class work easily when I put my mind to it, she commented. "Once he learns to attend," she concluded, "there will be no limits to his achievement!" Her conclusion was hopeful, and I wish I remembered her. "Brett has really tried since our conference to be more 'with it,'" she explained, "and has succeeded most of the time. I think he'll do well next year: the serious natural-scientist Brett will be more and more evidenced as he matures." Though "extremely bright," I apparently remained distracted by the world happening around me outside the classroom. Clearly, I was a nightmare of a student, but I appeared to have been immunologically healthy.

One year later, my next teacher relayed the following: "He is very capable but needs his energies channeled. Again, Brett is quick to grasp new concepts but his concentration span is short." She concluded: "He is happy and loving and has good retention of knowledge." In June 1974, yet another teacher from Marin Terrace wrote in her final evaluation: "He is a good worker and a rapid learner when his interest is aroused." In her estimation, I was a "lively, fun-loving boy," but, given what I remember of my childhood on Mount Tamalpais, how could I have been anything else? I was a blond-headed urchin, the carefree spawn of hippie parents in Mill Valley, running in white underpants through the wheat fields of Montana, over the beaches of California, and through the forests of the Sierra Nevada and the Cascades of the Pacific Northwest. I was healthy and loving, but there is no mention anywhere in the Marin Terrace documents of an underdeveloped immune system. I knew nothing but sunshine in those California days.

In the fall of 1975, however, I transferred to Cascade Elementary School in Montana after my father quit his job at Westinghouse. He had enrolled in law school at Lewis and Clark College in Portland; and while he looked for a house, my brother, mother, and I lived in Cascade with my grandparents. As in Mill Valley, I remember only flashes of my time in Cascade, including the one I alluded to earlier. I also remember cleaning and dismantling the old Quonset building with my grandfather while he secretly killed himself with cigarettes. "It'll be our secret, Brett," he had said. I have a distinct snapshot of him at this precise moment: he is to my left, and I have turned my head to look at him; he is backlit by the sun, so I see only a silhouette of the man. My brother, Aaron, was probably there, but I do not remember.

School in Cascade proved jarring for many reasons, not the least of which was that I had not learned cursive writing at Marin Terrace. When I was asked to write in cursive style by my elementary school teacher and could not, I was deeply embarrassed, to the point of tears. Marin Terrace had been Montessori-like, a less structured environment where teachers encouraged students to get "with it" by exploring the world on their own. It was a school where I could be "lively" and "fun-loving," characteristics my teacher had celebrated. The Mill Valley School District had opened Marin Terrace in 1957 because of the postwar baby boom. By 1962, the little school boasted some 300 students. However, in 1978, after the number declined to 141 students, the school district closed that slice of happy-go-lucky educational paradise. Since that time, the physical structure has gone through several iterations; as of this writing it houses the private Marin Horizon School. It turned out that Cascade Elementary School marched to a different pedagogical drummer.

"Brett has had a rather trying time learning to accept a structured type of school program," my Cascade teacher observed that fall. "Because Brett was having difficulties in reading he has been in a remedial reading group." I remember this about school in Cascade: the only thing I looked forward to was the prospect of riding a snowmobile to school, a promise my uncle

Lee baited me with, no doubt bribing me to study more. I also relished hunting around the farm, which I spent countless hours doing. In Cascade, my "citizenship" was rock solid, my teachers explained; my subject grades were "satisfactory minus" across the board. I see now, looking back carefully into my past, that the move to Montana constituted a major life waypoint for me. No more climbing the red-limbed Pacific madrones of Mount Tamalpais, spending hours exploring the forest. No more sliding down its steep, grassy sides on cardboard boxes with Taschi, the lovely collie-coyote mix, running behind me, tail wagging. No more skipping around on the soft-sand beaches near Mill Valley. No more *To Our Children's Children's Children* on reel-to-reel, the Moody Blues soundtrack of my Mill Valley youth. The return to Montana was cold and raw, as only Montana can be. There were nights when Aaron and I were warned to leave my mother alone as she tended her dying father. I was further disillusioned by school and became even less engaged. The move away from Mill Valley represented the slow disintegration of my family as my parents careened uncontrollably toward divorce. Taschi quietly walked away one day and never returned. We stapled posters of her to telephone poles, but nobody ever responded. "She was part wild animal, Brett," my mother explained. "She went away to die alone." Within the decade, my father left my mother, brother, and me, essentially to practice law out of his Volvo, and nothing would ever be the same again.

While hunting the feral tonalities roaming in the recesses of my mind, and carefully luring my memories into the cages of words, what I did learn when looking back at my time in Cascade is that my relationship to Montana became an enduring part of how I viewed myself during my childhood. As cold and gray as the winter of 1975–76 was, it was burned onto my soul, not unlike the way the tips of frostbitten fingers turn black and burn with pain when cold. I do not have to look far into my memories to see elk hunting with my grandfather near Lincoln, for example, and a cold Remington Model 30, the "meat gun," as my family calls this mythic rifle, resting across my lap when I was eight years old. "Just wait here, Brett. They'll come," he whispered. They never did, but it was so quiet after the last words had slipped from his lips in the form of small clouds that evaporated into the cold evening air. I watched him disappear into the woods, his own rifle resting in the crook of his arm. I had never felt so completely alone as a young boy, stolen away from the California warmth; but I also knew I could be nowhere else. The Helena National Forest is a big place for an eight-year-old boy, even one with a rifle. But those two or three hours seared themselves into my memory for some reason. Just as frostbitten hands will always be sensitive to the cold, my soul will always be sensitive to Montana. When I cross into Montana airspace, I feel it.

Writing about his Montana childhood in *This House of Sky*, Ivan Doig recalled that his memories began with his mother's death on his sixth birthday. "The remembering begins out of that new silence," he wrote. "Through the time since, I reach back along my father's tellings and around the urgings which would have me face about and forget, to feel into these oldest shadows for the first sudden edge of it all." As it does for most souls from Montana, remembering for Doig begins with landscape. "It starts," he explained, "early in the mountain summer, far back among the high spilling slopes of the Bridger Range of southwestern Montana." Leeward of his mother's last breath, he saw "just a single flicker," but the landscape, the colossus around him, welded together memories in the form of an epic story. "Memory is a set of sagas we live by, much the way of the Norse wildmen in their bear shirts," he explained. Doig told his story with the intensity of a Norse berserker battling other men, as if possessed by the demon of remembrance; but he, too, remained flummoxed by the unevenness of memory's terrain, which resembles ruts baked into an old Montana hunting road. Memory, with its "eddying but detailed power," exists inside us but almost independently of us. "If," he mused, "somewhere beneath the blood, the past must beat in me to make a rhythm of survival for itself—to go on as this half-life which echoes as a second pulse inside the ticking moments of my existence—if this is what must be, why is the pattern of remembered instants so uneven, so gapped and rutted and plunging and soaring?" Doig concluded that childhood memories resemble childhood itself, "a most queer-lit and shadow-chilled time." Existing in the "near-neighborhood of dreams," memory is "almost as casual with its hospitality," coming and going as it pleases, which is what makes trapping it in cages of words so complicated.

This proved particularly true of words used to describe family memories. These "blood words," Doig observed, though "plain packets of sound like any other," are critical to telling our story because they "speak to the mysterious strengths of lineage." This is the voice of family history, perhaps more aptly called blood history, which tracks us from generations past. Doig wrote, "I admit the marvel that such sounds are carried to us from the clangs and soughs of tongues now silent a millennium into the past, calling on and on, in their way, like pulses of light still traveling in from gone stars." This is what history is: the organized stories, "like pulses of light still traveling in from gone stars," that we keep with us; and though we cannot always control their comings and goings, they give us waypoints if we take the time to scan the horizon. "This set of sagas, memory," he noted, "over and over self-told, as if the mind must have a way to pass its time, docket all the promptings for itself, within its narrow bone cave." But rehearsing history, family or otherwise, is about more than the mind devising ways to "pass its time." Rather, it is about the mind fathoming ways to comprehend and plot, through remembered patterns, its present situation and possible futures. In a way, history is all that we have to navigate by.

Doig disliked school in Montana, much like I did. "School struck me as a kind of job where you weren't allowed to do anything," he wrote. "I had free time in my head by the dayfull, and spent it all in being lonesome for ranch life and its grownups and its times of aloneness." That is how I remember much of my childhood as well, "being lonesome for ranch life." After my father moved the family to Portland, we still traveled to Montana every summer to help with the harvest at the Cascade farm. When we left Montana at the end of every summer, when the harvest was over and the air felt crisp with the coming hunting season, I often returned to Portland with artifacts from the farm. And they grew bigger as I grew older. At first they were cat skulls, deer antlers, raccoon tails, beehives, and a lever-action Daisy BB gun; later, I dragged back an old green Kawasaki motorcycle with vice grips for a shifter, rifles, and then my grandfather's blue Ford pickup truck. At the same time that Janeway recovered from "serum sickness" and published his first articles on the clinical benefits of the intravenous use of the immunoglobulins, I surrounded myself with the material artifacts of Montana life. Montana became the epigenetic fiber of my identity; and even in high school, when I participated in Future Farmers of America, I always figured that my life and farming would converge once again. I was lonely for farm life every day but, importantly for this book, immunologically healthy.

— · —

Truth claims in memoir and history can be tricky business, but historians need to reacquaint themselves with such thresholds of evidentiary reality. Even before what some call the "post-truth presidency" of Donald J. Trump, memoirist Mary Karr had detected a "strange cynicism about truth" in American culture, one that had "permitted us to accept all manner of bullshit" from just about everybody, including memoir writers. Setting aside the political dangers of a citizenry that does not hold politicians accountable for truth-telling, this slip into a relativistic abyss—one where personal "experience," true or not, outweighs empirical "reality"—poses many dangers to our collective cultural health. Many readers, Karr has concluded, have determined that the "line between fiction and nonfiction is too subtle for us to discern," which has set up memoir writing for some serious recollecting skullduggery, including people just making things up. This has blurred the line between memory and facts about one's life—or anybody else's life, for that matter. When it comes to sheer entertainment, it is really not all that important if people embellish reality; but when it comes to discerning my family history, one that is meant to trace the emergence of a serious medical condition, the truth in my past becomes more important; otherwise it is not valuable. I cannot evade the notion that a true description can be retrieved from out there in the past, one that elucidates the appearance of my CVID. I have always looked to the past to understand truths in the world. The limiting factor is not truth itself but rather the evidence available to retrieve it.

Karr has correctly argued that in the United States a collective skittishness about making truth claims has metastasized, one that has gummed up the gears of our "collective moral machinery." She wrote, "I think a screw has come loose in our culture around notions of truth, a word you almost can't set down without quotes around it anymore." She continued: "Sometimes it strikes me that even when we know something's true, it's almost rude to say so, as if claiming a truth at all . . . threatens someone else's experience." Karr made the case in memoir writing for something she calls "reality," and for the memoirist's need to retrieve it as well as possible. That is why I often use the word *retrieve* when I talk about my family history of illness; because as much as I am crafting it, I also understand that something actually happened. And I seek to retrieve it, not make it up. History is intensively creative, but not fashioned from thin air.

If evidence existed of chronic infections in my childhood, then my CVID might have been congenital, something I have carried with me, to one degree or another, from my breast-milk-deprived infancy. But I was a healthy child, not even a little sickly. The truth of my family history of illness must lie elsewhere, then. Simply, either exposures and events happened later in my life that triggered my hereditary predisposition for CVID, or I had no hereditary predisposition and environmental factors alone caused the disease. This is the truth of my early childhood, at least for the purposes of this book.

CHAPTER 4

Proteins

I SIT DOWN TO WRITE THIS MORNING AND I DO NOT FEEL
well. I have managed to catch a cold and it has moved into
my sinuses and throat. I am plugged solid and have a headache;
my throat is sore and I have a rattling cough. I probably picked
something up at the hospital while receiving my immunoglobulin infusion. Patients at the Bozeman Health Cancer Center
sometimes arrive sick because of immunosuppressant med-
ications, usually for autoimmune disorders such as ulcerative
colitis or Crohn's disease, but they also weaken from chemotherapy. It is this specific kind of flu-like illness that resurrects
dark memories for me, particularly of what I now think was the
gradual emergence of my CVID. Judging from the conclusions
of the previous chapter, and my personal perception of my own
health, I think my white blood cells slowly stopped producing
antibodies, that it was not some shock to my body that suddenly
stopped their production. These memories of the deterioration

of my health are crisper than scenes from my childhood, because they come from the last decade; but as a diagnostic tool to better explain my illness, they also require more chronological and descriptive precision, so narrating them presents a series of fresh challenges. They are fresher memories, but they are also less mine, in a way that is hard to explain—the reality is that I share them with my illness.

Today, the Cancer Center serves as the modern umbilical cord through which I receive the passive supplemental immunity of the generous blood donors for CSL Behring, manufacturer of Privigen Immune Globulin Intravenous. It allows me to avoid being preyed upon by the daily onslaught of bacterial micropredators, such as my archnemesis, *Haemophilus influenza*—the tiny Khan in my life. This modern umbilical cord connects me to industrialized medicine in an intimate way, essentially making my body a cyborglike extension of Big Pharma. Botanist Hope Jahren, who worked in a University of Minnesota pharmacy preparing IV bags while in graduate school, understood the nature of this connection between human and machine. She observed that with intravenous medication, the "nurse cleans your skin, inserts a needle, and then leaves it there for hours, effectively making the needle, the tube, and the entire bag that is attached to it an extension of your vein—and all the liquid in the bag becomes an extension of your bloodstream." Indeed, while I receive my monthly IV dose of immunoglobulins, my body is linked not just to rubber hoses and bags but to an entire industrial system of blood production, one that flows throughout my whole body.

The last time I was linked to this industrial system, the man receiving chemotherapy in the chair next to me had a bad cold. He was slight with silver hair, from Florida originally. He had moved to Bozeman two years earlier, following his son who had attended Montana State University. Like so many, he and his wife had taken a liking to southwest Montana and decided to stay. Clutching a wad of tissue in his hand to wipe his sniffling nose and watery eyes, he told me of his family's tradition of eating clam chowder and steamed lobster during the holidays; he orders the live lobster directly from the Northeast. The tradition started years ago during a holiday road trip to Maine, in his family's RV, where they happened on a restaurant serving chowder and lobster on Christmas Eve. They relished it so much that they made it a yearly occasion, even after moving to the Rocky Mountains, where lobsters are quite rare in the wild. As these last words left his lips, disappearing among the bells and peeps of finicky IV pumps, he rested his head against the brown vinyl reclining chair, turned away from me, and gazed out the window toward the Bridger Range, where a blanket of fresh snow had fallen in the past several hours. It is easy to get lost in thought in the Cancer Center; I often find myself adrift in my own mind, pondering my own fragile medical stasis. He wiped his nose again and then glanced at his IV pump and the small clear bag dangling from it. "It's so delicious," he said. "The best in the world . . . I mean the Maine lobster," he laughed. I laughed with him.

In the Minneapolis Specialty Infusion Center, where I received my immunoglobulin infusions immediately after my CVID diagnosis, I once heard a woman scream so loudly as they poked the catheter needle in her hand that it made my blood curdle. "Oh, that one's just terrified of needles," a nurse later explained. Initially, my infusion in Minneapolis took eight hours because of the slow pump rate, a precaution necessitated by my initial adverse reaction to the immunoglobulin treatment. I therefore had hours to burn while watching patients of all shapes and sizes walking—or wheeled in chairs or on gurneys by nurses—past my little infusion nook. I observed many gaunt, ashen bodies in Minneapolis, the bodies of very sick people, and I often wondered if mine looked that sickly, too. I had weighed only 150 pounds when I left the hospital in 2011, and I was putting on weight slowly. "Just let me know if you start losing more weight," my doctor had explained, worried about the possible appearance of lymphoma. I saw many children in the Specialty Infusion Center with PICC lines (a type of long catheter inserted into a large vein) dangling from their noodlelike arms, their beds surrounded by stuffed animals and other toys. I heard the sweet octaves of their voices venturing innocent questions just above the ever-present white noise of hospital equipment and medical chatter, usually asking about fruit juice choices, cookies, or how to work the television remote. They asked these questions nonchalantly, as IV pumps dripped medicines or platelets or blood or immunoglobulins into their desperate little bodies. The nurses were angels in these circumstances and always explained the juice and snack choices patiently.

Whatever bug I have caught at the moment, perhaps from the lobster-eating gentleman, I do not feel too awful, not yet anyway, but a mild infection has definitely taken root. I have not exhibited a fever: my Minneapolis doctor tells me that, if there is any sign of fever whatsoever, I am to call him immediately and probably begin a course of antibiotics. When I am not feeling well, I often become quiet, distracted, and melancholic, because I am reminded of the seriousness of my disease; I am reminded that I cannot fight even the simplest illnesses alone, and herein lies the finitude of my life. The packed, inflamed sinuses, the chunks of dark green phlegm I cough up, the uncomfortable sensitivity to cold and sharp sounds, the low energy—all this evokes in me visions and sensations of the gradual emergence of the disease that nearly killed me.

Frankly, the possibility of being prey to micropredatory bacteria terrifies me. It reminds me that my immune system, millions of years in the making, finely tuned to live on this green planet pulsing with microscopic life, has broken down and I have few defenses against microorganisms, other than those offered by the grace of modern medicine. In a world before Charles Janeway I would be dead. David Quammen, who has written on large and small predators alike, has observed that "exterminating all alpha predators is basic to the enterprise of civilization," and I agree; but I would add that keeping micropredators at bay has been equally as important for the success of modern civilization, particularly after the advent of germ theory and antibiotic chemotherapy. My vulnerability to bacteria makes me feel exposed and left behind, a half-man in a world that demands evolutionarily advanced whole ones.

In 1881, when Élie Metchnikoff, a Russian zoologist, first pondered the existence of cells dedicated to the defense of the body, he framed the immune system in the language of nineteenth-century legal and political thought. Think about it: the immune system is seen as the body's defense against a dangerous outside world. Metchnikoff saw the body as similar to the nation, and the nation as similar to the body—both are in the business of self-preservation through the defense of borders. While observing the cells of transparent starfish larva under a microscope, he wrote, "It struck me that similar cells might serve in the defense of the organism against intruders." And so his quest to better understand the body's immune defenses began. Historian Ed Cohen argued that our understanding of the immune system is therefore a "biopolitical hybrid," one born from Metchnikoff's cellular observations and Thomas Hobbes's notions of "natural rights." This biopolitical nexus yielded "immunity-*as*-defense," wherein "defense is acknowledged for the first time as a capacity of a living organism," which transformed "how we imagine what it means to be a human living among other humans." The body defends itself from other people and their microorganisms. In the late nineteenth century, Metchnikoff's theories localized disease resistance as the activity of cells and molecules that guarded the frontier of the body's edge from foreign invaders.

This discrete body, one guarded by immunity-*as*-defense, became the epitome of the "modernized body." As Cohen described, the modernized body was informed by a constellation of historical forces, including "finance capital, philosophical reflection, and scientific theory, not to mention military formations, colonial relations, religious reformations, technological developments, kinship dynamics, industrial processes, educational regimes, health care protocols, among many other factors." Essentially, Cohen explained, the modernized body sought to "localize human beings within an epidermal frontier that distinguishes the person from the world for the duration which we call life." Cohen contrasted the modernized body to what philosopher and literary theorist Mikhail Bakhtin has called the medieval "grotesque body," one not neatly localized behind an epidermal frontier but "open to the world both temporally and spatially, simultaneously eating, shitting, fucking, dancing, laughing, groaning, giving birth, falling ill, and dying." This is the premodern body, one yet to be viewed as guarded by immunity-*as*-defense, one interacting fluidly with the world around it.

Cohen explained that with the formulation of immunity-*as*-defense, life became an endless challenge of "boundary maintenance," and the self became associated more with the material body within this guarded perimeter than with the soul, which had been a hallmark of medieval thinking. Cohen concluded that "biological immunity makes the body *modern*." But if Cohen is correct, then what does this make my immune-compromised body? I would die if a catheter needle did not pierce my epidermal frontier monthly, penetrating my veins and injecting immunoglobulins manufactured by other bodies into my bloodstream. In this manner, my body becomes less an example of the localized modern body, with its immunity-*as*-defense, than a globalized immunity-*as*-commons body, one formed with the aid of other bodies, ones not even living near me, and then synthesized by industrial medicine. I have come to see my body as less modern than postmodern in this regard: nationless, borderless, as porous as Swiss cheese, and dependent, like the "grotesque body" of the medieval age, one interacting fluidly with the world around it.

But the medicine my porous body receives through its epidermal frontier does not always work for me. This morning, my physical symptoms have occurred at multiple sensory levels, and they prove far better at triggering memories than my active self-reflective remembering does. When I get sick the memories become intense, because there is a physical association with my memories: they are more than simply disembodied scenic spirits, or the ghosts of "talk-story," as Maxine Hong Kingston refers to memories in her *Woman Warrior*. They are embodied and physically real: they are part of what Charles Sherrington called "the material me." My memories of illness are a physiological manifestation of pathological phenomena, ascending from my visceral and external sensory experiences to become the biological material of my mind and body. I now know they are all interconnected—my body, my memories, my disease, my history, and now my medicine.

I do not remember precisely when my CVID symptoms started, but I think they started gradually, over the course of a couple of years. One early episode that stands out occurred in Japan in May 2006, while I was traveling to the city of Mina-mata, the location of a deadly methylmercury-pollution event that occurred in the mid-twentieth century and which served as the centerpiece of my book on Japan's modern environmental calamities. I had just arrived by bullet train at the Nagoya Station and was standing at the center of a crowded atrium, contemplating whether to get something to eat before I ventured to my hotel. Thousands of people swirled around me in every direction as they made their way through the station. Suddenly, I started to feel disoriented and confused, displaced from my own body. My vision grew increasingly cloudy and darker, and I immediately moved to a less congested corner of the station, where I sat down on the floor. But my condition did not improve. I went into a small *tonkatsu* restaurant, thinking that a bite of breaded pork might help; but my disorientation persisted, and I decided to slowly make my way toward my hotel, where, after checking into my room, I rested for several hours.

I debated going to the hospital in Nagoya, but as I slowly gained control over my wits, I decided against it. The next morning I felt better, but anxious: I had never felt anything like that before. What had happened to me? It was as if a switch had been flipped. As I thought about the episode over the next several days, I concluded that it must have been an anxiety attack of some kind; but in retrospect, as I think about the causal chain in my family history of illness, I see now that it may have portended much more, perhaps something stemming from my body's inability to regulate the microorganisms in my gastrointestinal and respiratory tracts. Did something in my plasma cells switch at this moment, so that they suddenly began producing fewer and fewer antibodies in response to bacterial invasion? Was it possible to feel such a thing happen in my body? Was a switch or blockage of this nature discernable by other parts of the body, such as the central nervous system and the brain? Or, conversely, was the anxiety itself symptomatic of a micro-predator rebellion under way in my body, one sending complex signals to my central nervous system? My hypothesis now, after having lived with CVID for half a decade, is that I might also have had an inner ear infection, a common symptom of CVID, and that it made me extremely dizzy and lightheaded, because I have experienced the same sensations since, sometimes while teaching.

The same year as my Nagoya trip, I visited Bozeman Health Deaconess Hospital on several occasions with strange tingling sensations in my face, particularly around my mouth and throat. I was sure it was related to my anxiety problems. My doctor referred me to an ear, nose, and throat specialist, and I had several examinations of my throat and mouth. When the specialist discovered nothing, he ordered an MRI of my brain to determine if a tumor was causing the irritating sensations in my face. The radiologist, too, saw nothing. My doctor thought that I might need antianxiety medication, and he prescribed one; but it made me feel cloudy, dull-witted, and slow, so I immediately stopped taking it, despite his advice that I continue. The facial sensations persisted for a year or two, and stopped around the same time as my immunological collapse and the beginning of my immunoglobulin replacement therapy.

What I remember about this phase in my life is the gradual realization that I lived in a vulnerable and penetrable body, one that made itself known to me through its increasing microbial porousness. I was sick all the time. I stopped touching doorknobs. I rarely shook hands. I kept meetings with students to a minimum. I drank truckloads of orange juice. Simultaneously and unconsciously, I began to research and write, in my professional capacity as a historian, about bodily pain caused by pollution in Japan. Unbeknownst to me, I had started to rehearse in the pages of my books an autobiography of the discomfort within "the material me," even though I was not the actual research topic. In my book *Toxic Archipelago*, I formulated the hypothesis that bodily pain caused by environmental toxins ranging from cadmium poisoning to methylmercury poisoning alerts people to their physical place in the natural world. I had not yet recognized it, but I was slowly becoming alerted to my place in the world's bacterial and viral ecosystems, particularly the ones dwelling in and around my body. Contorted and diseased Japanese bodies served as proxies for my growing awareness of my diseased body. These signals came from inside my own physical self, and they poured onto the pages of my historical writing. I just did not yet know how to interpret them.

Then, it happened. Within about a year of the Nagoya incident, I started waking up every morning feeling awful: painful headaches, inflamed and throbbing sinuses, infected upper respiratory tract, chronic diarrhea and irritable bowels, aching sore throat, chills and shivers, eyes welded shut from conjunctivitis, sensitivity to cold and loud noises, periodic night sweats, and fever. One evening, I leaned over the bathroom sink, looked into the mirror, and splashed my face with warm water. I blew my nose into my wet hands and saw that my hands were splattered red with blood. Nothing new there; but as I looked up into the mirror, a green liquid with the consistency of waffle batter, intermixed with stripes of red blood, began draining out of my nose. To my amazement, it drained for close to half a minute. By the time my sinuses had drained, about a quarter cup of the green-and-red discharge had accumulated in my hands and in the sink. I was terrified. "What the hell is happening to me?" I thought. "This was inside my fucking head?" It was like I always had the flu. My body constantly ached. The mornings were always the worst: the association with bodily pain and mornings became so pronounced that I feared going to bed at night, wondering what new bodily secretion and pain the morning would bring.

The mornings blended into one continuous painful and secretory bodily experience: The alarm rings and I pull myself from the bed, quickly putting on something warm. I am shivering. My pajamas are drenched. I go into the bathroom, lean over the sink, and cough up dark green phlegm until my throat is raw. Seeking sinus relief, I try to blow it out of my nose, but I never again experience the sheer relief of the green batter draining from my perennially infected head. I assume it lives in there permanently now. The more I cough, the longer my voice will remain hoarse for the rest of the day, making it hard to lecture in the classroom. I place a towel over my back and lean against the heater element in the bathroom, warming myself. Next, I have to tend to my eyes, which are glazed shut from discharge. I wipe them clean with a warm washcloth and then dump several drops of Clear Eyes into them, so I can be presentable at work. I then step into the hot shower, even though I have a strong revulsion to getting wet. The sound of the water irritates me, too. Finally, after taking two or three ibuprofen to blunt the body aches, and putting the remainder of the bottle in my pocket, I prepare to drive to work.

The winter months in Montana proved the most difficult because just sitting in my truck, waiting for the heater to warm the cab, made my body ache. If Montana created my mental profile during that critical winter of 1975–76, after my family had left Mill Valley to witness my grandfather's death at the Cascade farm, then Montana would eventually kill me, too, in some future winter, the shiny blade of its cold piercing my defenseless body.

Starting in 2007, I also went through a divorce. About the time that my symptoms began to worsen, I left my wife and house and moved into a friend's basement. When I told my mother, she drove the next morning from Anacortes to see me. "You look awful," she said, stepping from her car. "Christ's sake, Brett." I also lived for a spell with my friend Michael. I had been elected department chair in 2005, so I was working long hours in the office. Often, I just pulled out a sleeping bag and slept there. Once, Jonathan, a cool, silver-haired janitor, peered down at the sleeping bag on my office floor and quipped, "That's not good, dude." I spent most my time at work worrying about my conjunctivitis, wondering why, even after getting antibiotic drops, it continued to glaze my eyes shut. Whenever I took antibiotics, I would feel better for a spell, but then, when I finished the prescribed course, the symptoms just returned, often more pronounced.

I see that my immune system had probably collapsed, or had at least partially collapsed, in the winter of 2007—two years after I became department chair, after I had started my divorce and while I was living in various basements. It is a disorienting feeling to lose the ability to fight anything, all bodily shields compromised. It is disorienting to be a giant compared to your predator and yet completely unable to defend yourself. I have never fully trusted my body again, which is why being sick, as I am now, while I write, frightens me. At the time, somebody suggested it might be my tonsils. One friend suggested that it was workplace stress. Was it the divorce proceedings? Was it the Nagoya incident? On February 24, 2008—my forty-first birthday—I received a generous full-professor job offer from Yale University and divorce papers from my ex-wife's lawyer, who, I learned, had a shark tank in his office. I was under an enormous amount of stress, and it kept mounting. In many respects, my life had unraveled before my crusted eyes, and as the stress spooled up, so did the incremental deterioration of my health. My decision-making became more definitive and slightly edgy. I started dating a friend in Minneapolis and found myself visiting her for the 2010 winter holiday. It was then that my health completely collapsed and I ended up in the University of Minnesota Medical Center. In retrospect, it all happened rather quickly, though it did not seem so at the time.

— · —

We all have existential waypoints in life, ones that determine, after we have experienced them, how we retrospectively describe our approaches to such waypoints and our future departures from them. Such waypoints impregnate the past and future events of our life with meaning, an invented teleological purposefulness. The Bolshevik takeover of Russia was Vladimir Nabokov's waypoint, guiding the bulk of his interpretation of his life before the communist takeover and after. The death of his wheezing mother in the Bridger Range, or perhaps the sheep drive near Cut Bank under the black clouds of a Montana electrical storm, created meaning in Ivan Doig's life. Likewise, the suffering of his mentally and physically ill mother drove Richard Wright's combative life. His telling of recognizing this waypoint is visceral and revealing. He explained, "My mother's suffering grew into a symbol in my mind, gathering to itself all the poverty, the ignorance, the helplessness; the painful, baffling, hunger-ridden days and hours; the restless moving, the futile seeking, the uncertainty, the fear, the dread; the meaningless pain and the endless suffering." The waypoint began guiding not just his approach to his mother's illness but also his departure from it, well after the event itself had disappeared abaft and he had started anticipating his future life. "Her life set the emotional tone of my life, colored the men and women I was to meet in the future, conditioned my relation to events that had not yet happened, determined my attitude to situations and circumstances I had yet to face." He wrote, "At the age of twelve I had an attitude toward life that was to endure, that was to make me seek those areas of living that would keep it alive, that was to make me skeptical of everything while seeking everything, tolerant of all and yet critical." These existential waypoints color everything that happens before and after them in the context of remembering, and my immunological collapse is one of those points. I take periodic existential bearings of it much as a coastal sailor takes bearings of a prominent rocky outcropping or an exposed reef.

The discovery of Catholic faith colored Thomas Merton's life, as did his entry into the Trappist monastery at Gethsemani in Kentucky. But it was his intellectual rejection of bourgeois individualism, the recognition of our entanglement in the sticky web of people and objects around us, the world that we are thrown into, which provided the waypoint that most redirected his life's purpose. This is the same reality that philosopher Martin Heidegger painted in his discussion of the person as "being-in-the-world," though Heidegger's realization of the human place in the world was not driven by the discovery of Catholic holism. Instead, it was the product of philosophical concepts such as "facticity" and "thrownness," concepts I discussed earlier but which are worth rehearsing briefly here. The family medical culture that discouraged breastfeeding and encouraged mothers to use formula was part of the milieu of my life, but so were Janeway's clinical and research accomplishments and his identification of CVID and the use of immunoglobulin replacement therapy. These are only part of the sticky web of people and things that I live within as a "being-in-the-world." I was thrown into them and can do little to control them.

But part of the world I was thrown into was also a microbial one, a bony reef of microorganisms that eventually overwhelmed my body. They and the signals they caused and sent also became part of the world I was thrown into, as was the genetics of my family background. I can do little about "the material me" in this regard, other than perhaps eat more yogurt. By contrast, Merton's account of his life is a transcendent "autobiography of faith," a rejection of "the material me" in favor of the composite souls that enter and exit our life. He recognized that, "since no man ever can, or could, live by himself and for himself alone, the destinies of thousands of other people were bound to be affected, some remotely, but some very directly and near-at-hand, by my choices and decisions and desires, as my own life would also be formed and modified according to theirs." Context, too, mattered for Merton, but in a metaphysical rather than physical way. He pondered the immaterial me; I ponder the material one.

In some respects, as I reflect on my life, remembering and rendering my story depends on two navigational waypoints, both of which color the entirety of my life. They made me aware of my own place in the world. The first is the winter of 1975–76 in Montana, where I attended Cascade Elementary School as my grandfather died; the second is the collapse of my immune system, and the inception of my awareness that my life occurs within a porous and vulnerable body and unfolds within the historically constructed world around me. The winter of 1975–76 in Montana determined the tenor of so much of my later adolescence in Portland, transforming me into an often melancholic, unengaged, and quiet kid. I remember being, in Portland, in a largely internalized world, never able to fully understand how to externalize my thoughts.

Most of my memories from these years are of events that occurred outside, either skiing in the Cascades or boating on

Oregon's lively coastal streams. I remember an epic canoe trip down the North Santiam River, above Mill City, where my father was seriously injured. "You don't want to take that thing down this stretch of river, I assure you," one of the three men in kayaks had explained as the three Walker boys prepared to launch our canoe into the North Santiam's swift current. Some years earlier, my father had bought an old silver Alumacraft canoe, the last boat any experienced paddler would want to take down white-water rapids. But this canoe saw a great deal of action before my brother finally wrapped it around a rock in the Clackamas River. In this stalwart seabird, we had nearly killed ourselves in the Smith River, near White Sulphur Springs, Montana. We had also nearly drowned in the Blackfoot River near Lincoln. In the frothing water and eddying currents of the North Santiam, my brother and I looked like ruffled grouse in our shorts and bright orange life vests—we spent most of the day in the water, not on the water, just two little white heads bobbing down the rapids. The excursion came to an abrupt halt when my father followed the boat off the Mill City Falls, slamming the sharp stern of the aluminum canoe into one of his testicles. He barely got ashore with his life. I remember looking through the driver's window into the blue Volvo to see my father with his shorts off and one swollen red testicle resting gingerly on his lily-white inner thigh. After we arrived back in Portland, the swollen monster was surgically removed, but the experience did not quell my desire for a childhood spent kayaking and canoeing on many of the Northwest's finest white-water streams, particularly while I was in high school.

After my family moved to West Linn, a suburb of Portland, I transferred yet again, this time to Sunset Elementary School. I continued to be disengaged from school. Our West Linn house had a glorious view of the Cascades, and I recall watching the

1980 eruption of Mount Saint Helens. I entered West Linn
High School in 1981 and continued to earn lackluster grades.
The only classes I found interesting were Agricultural Business
Management, Agricultural Production, and Forestry and Wild-
life Management, because I saw these courses as part of my
roadmap back to Montana and the Cascade farm. They came
closest to externalizing my internal nostalgia for Montana and
for being on the farm with my grandfather's ghost. In West
Linn, I discovered beer, pot, cars, friends, sex, and everything
a young man does in high school; but I continued to live on
the margins of high school life. I spent nearly every weekend
ski racing at Mount Hood, which in retrospect probably saved
me from the drug-infested dustbin of a wasted middle-class life.

I played junior varsity baseball at West Linn High School
and was nearly beaned by a Mitch Williams fastball during
practice. I played soccer as well, but mainly as part of dry-land
training for ski racing. Nothing in school engaged me at an
intellectual level, mainly, I see now, because of my myopic fan-
tasies about Montana life. I took history classes, but they failed
to pique my curiosity whatsoever. Words on the page had no
flavor for me; only actual things outside did—things like skulls,
bones, bullets, engines, and farm tools. It was material objects,
the ones I found outside, that I could touch, that made me
fantasize. I did not read books from school but instead raised
broiler chickens in our suburban backyard. I weighed them
daily, keeping track of them for one of my classes. When it was
time to slaughter them, my teacher taught me how to cut the
bottom out of a bleach bottle and nail it upside down to a wall.
I then pulled a chicken's head through the spout, wedging the
body in the bleach bottle so it could not flap around, and then
cut its head off with a pocketknife, the kind with a fork and
spoon on the sides. I removed their limp, bloody bodies from

the bleach bottle and briefly boiled them in water over a Coleman camp stove to aid in removing the feathers. My father, who had left the house by this time, was horrified at what I was doing; my mother, a farm girl at heart, thought my fledgling chicken-raising skills might be useful and praised the effort even as she pulled pieces of feathers from her mouth during several spindly-chicken dinners together.

It was about 1982 that my parents separated. "I want to take you both to dinner," my father had said to Aaron and me one night. I knew it was coming. My parents fought relentlessly, and Aaron and I often listened to the intense bickering from the downstairs family room. When my father graduated from law school, he became more aloof. On this night, he took his two boys down the hill to Round Table Pizza and told us that he was separating from our mother, and that he was moving out of the house. By my reckoning, he was then gone from my daily life, and I saw him only on weekends during ski season. I do not remember him packing bags or even waving good-bye. It probably happened while Aaron and I were in school and Mom was at work at Nordstrom.

He still came by the house periodically, usually to work in the garage. He had several projects scattered throughout the garage. In one of my father's most notorious projects, he had begun accumulating antique woodworking tools at the house — such as wooden mallets and lathes — and had even priced teak lumber, in order to build a Seabird Yawl, a beautiful sailboat, in our driveway. I remember when he excitedly rolled out the blueprints for the craft — designed by Thomas Fleming Day — in front of me, expounding the virtue inherent in building a wooden sailboat without power tools. Once he'd abandoned the boat project, he bought a purple, rusted-out 1963 Jaguar XKE that he hoped to restore. "It's the year I graduated from high school," he pronounced. He even bought a welder to repair its rusted undercarriage, through which you could see asphalt. I never saw the car run, because it broke down while my father was driving it to the house. But I have to admit, both projects completely captured my imagination, too, even though they never left their respective boxes, which was always my mother's principal complaint leveled against my father. For my mother, being a "doer" ranked among the highest human virtues, and my father was far more a thinker than a doer.

He left the house, but in the summer, after we stopped traveling to Montana, we still fixed up old cars, motorcycles, and bicycles together, which became a passion I have never been able to shake. I did all these things with my father after he left, but I did not know him well during these years. I think I visited his apartment once. Where I remember him being is his law office in Oregon City, where I sat across the desk from him while he confronted me about my awful grades. "Don't you want to go to college?" he asked. I did not want to go to college. I am not even sure I really knew what college was. I still lived in my dreamscape of the Cascade farm, riding in a Massey Ferguson with my dead grandfather, where learning to change the oil of a four-wheel-drive Versatile tractor, not reading good books or writing thoughtful prose, meant something to me. I liked oil on my hands. During my senior year, however, my father made me come to his office every day after school to do my homework and, eventually, to prepare an application for college. I recall writing my personal statement with him, talking about a childhood spent kayaking and fishing Oregon's rivers, not discussing any academic preparation whatsoever. In the end, my competitive skiing, not my piss-poor grades, earned me admittance into college.

When my father left, my mother assumed the bulk of the responsibility for raising my brother and me. My father popped in now and then to work on wooden yawls and classic cars, but it was my mother whom I remember waiting in her nightgown at the top of the stairs, confronting my brother or me about drinking beer, smoking pot, or just staying out late. She worked full time at the retailer Nordstrom and often was still at work when my brother and I got home from school. She usually worked late. We lived frugally during these years. We heated our house with a woodstove insert and even went out to cut our own firewood. It is not surprising that, when he bought the chainsaw some years earlier, my father had acquired an antique Husqvarna chainsaw, an enormous one. It was like a Volkswagen Beetle engine with a butter knife poking out of the end — but we still managed to cut wood with it. My mother had her hands full in those years with two young boys three years apart in age, growing up in a rural Portland suburb.

In many ways, the Montana winter of 1975–76, and my summers spent on the farm thereafter, indelibly colored my life throughout high school. I never thought about doing well in school and perhaps trying to get into a good university and be somebody important, because I remained too preoccupied with rehearsing farm life in my imagination. It was not as simple as just taking agriculture classes and driving a farm truck, either. Rather, I dressed in western clothes, wore a Montana belt buckle, hunted elk in Oregon's Blue Mountains, listened to Neil Young — hell, I even tried to talk like Neil Young — chewed tobacco, drove my grandfather's blue Ford pickup, and wore his white farm hat. I told my raptured friends stories of Montana life and brought a friend to Cascade one summer, just to prove to him that the Chestnut Valley paradise existed. But this internal obsession with Montana stunted me and retarded my personal growth. My senior year, my father gave me a copy of David James Duncan's *The River Why*, which constituted my first real engagement with a book without ballistics or fishing lure information. Since it was about fishing on Oregon's coastal streams, he reasoned the book might appeal to me, and it did. Slowly, I began to read, and the stories I encountered began to replace the farm dreamscape in my imagination. We had stopped traveling to the farm, and the Montana of my imagination began to fade and a broader view of the world, one encouraged by reading, thinking, and imagining, in time replaced it.

"The material me" being formed in these years, and presently being remembered while I write this book, was an amalgam of experiences, many of which I preserved in memory. But many I did not, and family members have reminded me of them. What are memories in a physical or material sense that some are recalled and others are not? I witnessed all my experiences, but I remember only some of them. Do memories have the same physical nature as antibody proteins, and can they, also like antibody proteins, disappear? Of all the scenes that have passed before my eyes during my life, why does the silhouette of my grandfather at the Quonset hut in 1976 stand out so vividly? "It'll be our secret, Brett," he had said while he smoked his cigarette. Why did this scene endure the years while others did not? Similarly, why do I so vividly remember the disgusting scene of the green infectious batter draining out of my nose?

I recall the frightened look on my face in the mirror. I remember the shape of the mirror, and its cheap, peeling chrome frame. Our life stories, our histories, whether individual or shared, can only be built from the "tonalities" we remember, so the physical architecture of remembering, just like the cultural process of crafting histories, is critical to constructing a narrative of my family history of illness. But there is even more to remembering than our physical architecture, because our feelings, behaviors, and memories also spring from the bidirectional communication that occurs between the body's microbial communities and the visceral body and brain. In this way, my illness, or more specifically, the microbial blooms that infected my body, and which communicated with my body while they were killing me, represent the real composite that is "the material me," not just who I was then, but how I remember myself and the experiences that unfolded around and within me.

— . —

Constructing a biological architecture of consciousness and memory is the central concern of a memoir by Nobel laureate Eric Kandel. If my waypoints in life were the Montana winter of 1975–76 and my immunological collapse in 2010, then Kandel's was the Nazi takeover of Vienna and his family's flight to the United States, where he became a neuroscientist at some of the finest universities in the country. "Consciousness is a biological process," he insisted, and the "human mind and spirituality originate in a physical organ, the brain." Nothing we experience consciously happens outside the physical reality of the flesh of our bodies and the material world around us. Not Heidegger's "being-in-the-world," thrown as she or he is into the milieu of a historically constructed life. Not self-consciousness, or the cobbling together of an identity based on important life experiences. Not the contextualizing of a serious disease such as CVID and trying to make sense of my life before and after diagnosis. Had I died of pneumonia in Minneapolis, it would have been the result of the absence of the antibodies needed to defend my body from dangerous bacterial microorganisms, not some spiritual possession. Similarly, our interpretation of the world around us is not an out-of-body experience; rather, it is an in-the-body experience, the product of the "enormous number, variety, and interactions" of nerve cells within the brain, and cells and organisms in the body's bacterial communities, working to produce what we understand to be our life.

Memory is a critical part of the biological tool kit that has made the human species successful as a knowledge-making, knowledge-using, and knowledge-remembering species. "It gives us a coherent picture of the past that puts current experiences in perspective," Kandel explained of memory. "Without the binding force of memory," he continued, our "experience would be splintered into as many fragments as there are moments in our life." If our brains did not have the capacity for memory, "we would have no awareness of our personal history," which builds human identity because we are the products of "what we learn and what we remember." Without the biology of memory, we would be nothing more than historyless zombies, roaming a world where everything is new and needs to be relearned, where no lessons can be heeded, and without the historical context of things and ideas. There would be no historical scaffolding on which to build our increasingly sophisticated lives, just present uncontextualized newness. Though philosopher Friedrich Nietzsche recognized the "capacity to live *unhistorically*" as a critical ingredient in happiness, what he saw as the ability to "settle on the threshold of the moment forgetful of the whole past" would force us to become senseless cave dwellers, feeling our way through the unknown caverns of life. The "chaotic inner world" of history often presents a burden, Nietzsche believed, a dangerous burden that plants the seeds of conflict. James Joyce spoke to this heavy burden in *Ulysses*, in the famous line "History . . . is a nightmare from which I am trying to awake." But it is a nightmare we must endure to be truly human. I am biased, to be sure, but I have always thought that people with no interest in history are buffoons. If remembering is key to the healthy functioning of human bodies, then surely it is key to the healthy functioning of human societies.

Uncovering the secrets of the biology of memory became the Holy Grail for researchers conducting brain studies in the early twentieth century. Sigmund Freud, the father of psychoanalysis, speculated that, in explaining the mechanisms of the mind, the abstract structure of psychology would someday yield to biological explanations, as the physical architecture and chemistry of the brain became better understood. Freud wrote, "We must recollect that all of our provisional ideas in psychology will presumably one day be based on an organic substructure," or the biological functioning of the brain. Six years later he wrote that, in the context of our description of the workings of the brain, the deficiencies would "vanish if we were already in a position to replace the psychological terms by physiological or chemical ones," something that neuroscience was on the cusp of doing in the first half of the twentieth century. During this period, neuroscience formulated three principles that became the bedrock of modern brain studies. The neuron doctrine, the first of these principles, holds that the nerve cell, or neuron, is the elementary building block and basic signaler of the brain. Such cells contain the DNA that determines both the cell's reproduction and what proteins it produces in the cytoplasm in order to maintain the body's everyday functioning. The second principle is the ionic hypothesis, which describes how "action potentials" function, or the journey of a cell's electrical signal to elsewhere in the body. The third principle, the chemical theory of synaptic transmission, describes the manner in which two neurons communicate with one another through neurotransmitters and receptor molecules. With neuroscience, nerve cells serve as the basic unit of neurological activity, including memory formation.

In the 1890s, Santiago Ramón y Cajal, a Spanish artist and neuroscientist, sought to determine the distinct shape of individual nerve cells, which had eluded biologists because of nerve cells' irregular shapes and the tangled cellular "forests" or "nets" that they built during the brain's lifetime. "Since the full forest turns out to be impenetrable and indefinable," Cajal reasoned, "why not revert to the study of the young wood, in the nursery stage, as we might say?" To isolate the "young wood," Cajal studied newborn, rather than adult, animal brains, which enabled him to see individual nerve cells, as well as their surface membranes, before complex neuronal forests had grown. In newborn brains, he explained, "nerve cells, which are still relatively small, stand out complete," and he identified the nerve cell's three main parts: the nucleus, a single axon, and the many dendrites. Cajal had illustrated the basic structure of the brain, and the interconnected forest that such neurons created became the key to understanding signaling between nerve-cell presynaptic terminals. With the work of Cajal, who received the Nobel Prize in 1906, neuroscience had reduced the brain to an organ composed of circuits with specific roles and signal directions, with sensory neurons sending stimulus from the outside world to the inside world of the brain's motor neurons.

Eventually, scientists determined that learning and memories are stored in the brain as actual anatomical changes in synaptic connections—the creation of new "forests" of neurons—either through the reinforcement of existing connections or the formation of new ones. Such learning is the product of external sensory stimulation, such as my grandfather sitting me down in the forest near Lincoln, with a rifle on my lap, and walking away. "Just wait here, Brett, they'll come," he had whispered. I had been scared. That precise moment, that stimulation of fear and heightened awareness of the darkening woods around me, created "functional transformations" and built particular "systems of neurons" that have enabled me to recall the experience even though it happened more than four decades ago. Early on, Cajal had seen these anatomical changes. He observed that "mental exercise facilitates a greater development of the protoplasmic apparatus and of the nervous collaterals in the part of the brain in use," leading to the "formation of new collaterals and . . . expansions." In 1948, the Polish neuropsychologist Jerzy Kornorski labeled this anatomical development brain "plasticity," which in the brain facilitates "permanent functional transformations[,] . . . in particular systems of neurons as a result of appropriate stimuli or their combination." My memories of my grandfather, and of the infected discharge pouring from my nose, and of the kind African American nurse in Minneapolis telling me of the "magic" medicine are not free-floating dreams, a version of René Descartes's res cogitans (a thinking mind or soul) independently floating in my bony cranium or in the heavens, even. Rather, they are new physical forests of neuronal dendrites, axons, and terminals, built from my real experiences. They are "the material me," or the neurological forests of my life. In this way, memory, the very spirit of our being and identity, is a material thing, not a spiritual abstraction, even though it often feels like one. Through collecting and organizing these individual neurological forests, history is constructed.

Kandel's scientific contribution was to expand Cajal's and Kornorski's notion of synaptic plasticity. Kandel wrote, "I presumed that different forms of learning give rise to different patterns of neural activity and that each of these patterns of activity changes the strength of synaptic connections in a particular way. When such changes persist, they result in memory storage." This plasticity was part of the molecular chemistry of the synapse, and it became part of his "reductionist approach to the study of learning and memory." Kandel and his colleagues discovered through experiments on sea snails that "learning leads to a change in the strength of synaptic connections—and therefore in the effectiveness of communication—between specific cells in the neural circuit that mediates the behavior." By "strength," Kandel meant the "long-term effectiveness of synaptic connections," the persistence of certain memories over others, and the nature of the experience that originally forged the connections.

Eventually, other neurologists determined that the storage of memories over long periods of time, as opposed to short-term storage, requires the synthesis of new proteins. Everyday experiences undergo two stages of storage in the brain: short-term memory storage requires that the synapse's function changes; but the actual anatomy of the brain, aided by protein synthesis, must change for long-term memory storage to occur. In other words, Kandel and his colleagues discovered the biological basis for who I am, why I harbor the memories that I do, and why they are uniquely mine. Kandel wrote that, because "each human being is brought up in a different environment and has different experiences, the architecture of each person's brain is unique." In my case, the presence of proteins made me who I am by means of long-term memory storage; but so did the absence of proteins, specifically immunoglobulins, because my weakened immune system allowed certain microorganisms in my gut and respiratory tract to play a more pronounced role in bidirectional communication with my central nervous system and brain.

Could something so big as memory and history depend on proteins, a basic building block of life? What a beautifully reductionist notion: that our memories, and the vast expansion of memories hidden in history, depend on something as simple as proteins. Surely, this is why the word *protein* comes from the Greek word *proteios*, which means "of first or primary importance." Kandel observed that "almost all of the proteins in the brain have relatives that serve similar purposes in other cells in the body," meaning there are intrinsic connections between my CVID and the way I identify and remember myself. How our bodies remember through the synthesis of a new protein in response to an external experience is not dissimilar to how our bodies fight bacteriological invaders: the cell makes a DNA-determined protein. In the case of long-term memory, the protein involved is CREB (cyclic AMP response element-binding protein). It sends signals through another protein, called a kinase, to the sensory nerve cell's nucleus in order to create the brain's anatomical change and memory. Kandel concluded that "in the brain as in bacteria, genes are also servants of the environment. They are guided by events in the outside world." As with the body's immune system, memory, too, is a product of epigenetic forces.

But it is not just my genes that are steering my body. The brain is also guided by interoception, or signals occurring inside the body, and the body's microbial dwellers, too, can send these interoception signals. In 1884, William James, a philosopher and psychologist, first speculated on the bidirectional communication between the inner visceral body and the brain when he focused on those emotional instances when a "wave of bodily disturbance of some kind accompanies the perception of the interesting sights or sounds, or the passage of the exciting train of ideas." Usually, people believe bodily waves to be the "manifestation" or "expression" of the feelings. But what if the opposite was true? What if the "perception of the interesting sights or sounds, or the passage of the exciting train of ideas," sparked a "wave of bodily disturbance," which then became feelings as the body communicated them to the brain? James argued that "*the bodily changes follow directly the* PER-CEPTION *of the exciting fact, and that our feeling of the same changes as they occur* IS *the emotion.*" In this regard, he was among the first philosophers to take aim at the Cartesian res cogitans, one separate from the material body. James submitted that "a purely disembodied human emotion is a nonentity," and that "emotion dissociated from all bodily feeling is inconceivable." As mentioned, Charles Sherrington labeled this embodied human emotion as "the material me." It was Sherrington who introduced the term *interoception* as well, in order to distinguish sensations emanating from the internal visceral body from external perceptions. Such visceral feelings from inside our bodies, including our guts and their microbial communities, constitute the building blocks of emotions, self-awareness, and cognition.

Today, the enteric nervous system, a complex web of neurons that governs the gastrointestinal system, is often referred to as a "second brain," because the neurotransmitters and signaling molecules so resemble the actual brain. Bidirectional communication between the gut and the brain not only ensures proper gastrointestinal function but also determines feeling states, motivation, and higher cognition and drives intuitive decisions. The notion of having a "gut feeling," it turns out, is more than simply an analogy. Certain stress-related symptoms, such as anxiety, are often closely related to gastrointestinal disorders, such as irritable bowel syndrome, illustrating the physiological pathway in the "microbiota-gut-brain axis." Moreover, infections in the body, caused by a compromised immune system, can conspire to alter central nervous system function and behavior, particularly cognitive abilities. This "interkingdom signaling" between microorganisms and a human body even modulates visceral pain perception, with certain probiotic microbes raising a person's pain threshold. As one neurologist wrote, when it comes to the body's bacterial communities, "they monitor us" and "we monitor them."

The body's microorganisms have the ability to modify brain function behavior, and they can do so through noninfectious and nonimmune routes as well, such as vagal pathways directly to the brain. Through complex cellular signals that are analogous to our body's own, microbes are in continuous communication with our nervous system via such neurotransmitters as serotonin. Since realizing that *Haemophilus influenza*, a common enough microorganism, nearly killed me, I have wondered the degree to which this and other infectious microbes living in my immune-compromised body have shaped my feelings, memories, behaviors, and choices. Something like 75 percent of the body's immune cells dwell within the gut's lymphoid tissue, most of them designed the keep the body's gut microbes under immunological control, so it is not surprising that gastrointestinal challenges plague CVID patients. The basic fact that the gut plays such an important role in the immune system reminds me that my recollections of the beginning stages of my CVID symptoms occurred at a time when I was not the only one contributing to my body's feelings—these microorganisms were, too. Historian Julia Adeney Thomas has speculated on the role these bugs might play in our historical lives, positioning the microorganisms in our bodies as a problem of scale for historians and introducing what might be called a microbiological turn in historical studies.

The gut's lymphoid tissue needs to be well fortified by immune cells because it confronts some one thousand separate species and some seven thousand separate strains of microbes, as well as 3.3 million nonhuman genes, some of which have the ability to penetrate lumen tissue barriers and cause infection. Diet alters microbial composition, which is why different people have different microbial communities. *Bacteroides* are more prevalent in diets high in fat and protein, for example, while *Prevotella* are more common in high carbohydrate diets. Moreover, the elderly have different gut compositions than young adults, suggesting that the body's bacterial community is constantly changing. But microbes directly drive the immune system: both the innate and the adaptive immune systems struggle to maintain a healthy stability throughout the inside surfaces of our intestines and colon, where our cellular bodies end and the ecological communities of our microbial guests begin. The me-microbe interface is critical for a healthy life, and when the immune system falters, then this interface becomes anarchistic, leading to not just infection and inflammation but also mood swings, poor choices, irregular behavior, and memory problems by altering the circulation of cytokines (cell signalers that affect the behavior of other cells). In this manner, the immune system transduces the effect of bacteria for the central nervous system and our brain's higher cognitive functions. Some refer to the body's bacterial communities as the "forgotten organ," given the critical role they play in cognitive functions.

The body's microbial content has been linked to autism spectrum disorders. Often, autistic children exhibit low levels of *Bacteroides fragilis*; and increasing the levels of the microbe in mice with autistic symptoms improved their behavior. Similarly, researchers have shown that bacteria such as *Lactobacillus* and *Bifidobacterium* reduce anxiety. Such bacteria also initiate biochemical and molecular changes, such as altered levels of corticosterone in the blood, which affects memory, and gene expression in BDNF (brain-derived neurotrophic factor), which is associated with Kornorski's brain plasticity. Mainly active in the hippocampus, cortex, and basal forebrain, BDNF is made up of proteins encoded with specific genes that encourage the growth and differentiation of new forests of neurons and synapses. These bacteria also alter neurotransmitter signaling in important ways. While their role is similar to the role that the body's microbial reef plays in immunological modulation during breastfeeding, such microbes are also an epigenetic component of higher brain function. Humans, as a history-making metazoan host, have coevolved with these microbes. They thrive in our bodies because of a ready supply of nutrients and stable ambient temperature, whereas our bodies depend on their enzymatic ability to digest food. But as it becomes clearer the degree to which our higher cognitive functions are assisted by the biochemical and molecular changes caused by these bacteria, we may discover that our interdependence runs deeper than that. It might be part of their evolutionary strategy to make us happier. As neurologist John Cryan wrote, "Happy people tend to be more social. And the more social we are, the more chances the microbes have to exchange and spread."

— · —

At this point, I have reached three conclusions about my family history of illness, ones born of an exploration of my Minneapolis hospitalization, Janeway's discovery of CVID, and a survey of my childhood and adolescence records and memories for signs of congenital or early onset immunological problems. In a sense, I have explored the category *illness* in my family history of illness by recounting my diagnosis, the 1952 identification of CVID, and the history of the immunoglobulin replacement therapies that have kept people like me alive. I have also unpacked the category *my* in this nagging sentence by exploring new medical theories of the body's microbial communities and how the body's microorganisms, the coral reef that is "the material me," contribute to the functioning of the immune system and the central nervous system, including creating certain behaviors and lasting memories. My internal viscera, and the microorganisms that call this reef home, contribute to the cognitive process of creating "me," my individual consciousness in the most material sense. They are contributors to my autobiography of disease in more ways than one.

To begin with, I did not have the congenital form of CVID, not even some relatively mild early-onset variety, during my childhood and adolescence. No evidence from my youth, whether in medical documents, in the form of absences from school, or stored in people's memories, suggests that I was a sickly child, a little runny-nosed runt more susceptible than other children to bacterial infections. I never once had pneumonia, meningitis, sepsis, or other life-threatening infections that plague children with seriously weakened immune systems. As my mother told me in the hospital after I started to recover, "Neither you nor Aaron was a sickly child. You just weren't, Brett."

I cruised the beaches of Northern California in my underpants, waded in the streams of the Sierra Nevada turning stones in search of crawdads, dined on dirt and drank creek water in the Cascade Mountains, and routinely swam, fished, and waterskied in Montana's lakes. I inadvisably played with bats in the old barn on the Cascade farm, befriended mangy stray cats, crudely tanned my own raccoon skins and then wore their rotting hides on my head, dangled reeking gopher tails from my Schwinn Stingray, boiled animal skulls and displayed them in my bedroom, cut my bare feet on shattered glass in the muddy sloughs and then had dogs lick my wounds clean (Grandma Frances always said this was the best remedy), and challenged my fledgling immune system in any number of routine child-hood ways. My immune system withstood all these challenges and many more, never once failing to produce antibodies in the face of bacteriological bad actors, as it later failed to do in Minneapolis.

My second conclusion is that I am certain my CVID appeared over the course of about four years, starting around 2006, and was accompanied by extreme stress at my work-place after I became department chair, and by anxiety at home around the time of my divorce. The pivotal set of events in my memory remains the anxiety attack at Nagoya Station in 2006 and the later trips to the hospital to find an explanation of the irritating facial sensations and other nervous-system symptoms. I do not remember being prone to infections whatsoever before 2006, before I was department chair. I had traveled extensively around the world, living in Japan for years at a time, and I never had problems with persistent infections while abroad, even while living among unfamiliar bugs. Looking back at these four critical years between 2006 and 2010, I see now that as my body produced fewer and fewer immunoglobulins, an unbalanced communicative loop occurred between the increasingly unruly microbial communities in my gastrointestinal tract and my cen-tral nervous system, affecting my behavior and moods. I know this because of the onset of routine diarrhea and gastrointestinal problems, and the spontaneity of my choices. I recall this in my chronic depression during these years, in my mood swings, in my ways of remembering these events and, most importantly, in my writing, which became eerily focused on bodily pain. I did not know it at the time, but I had started to write my own story, through the experiences of others.

My third conclusion is that my obsession with farm life in Montana was probably more than just simple boyish nostalgia. I now see that it was about family and landscape. For reasons that remain unclear to me, I was drawn to the Cascade farm and my dead grandfather in ways that go beyond simple youthful yearning and that beg questions about the power of blood affinities to drive "the material me." When my grandfather eased that insulin needle into his stomach while we sat together his truck, was his body speaking to mine in a language beyond words, in a way that only Doig's "blood words" can? Was he speaking to me in that way when he coolly said, "It'll be our secret, Brett," in Great Falls in a hushed voice months before his death? What secret was he talking about? "Why 'our' secret, Grandpa?" I want to ask. I thought he was talking about his smoking, and he probably was, but maybe his blood words penetrated much deeper than either of us could possibly know. Just as "the material me" is affected by the microorganisms that inhabit my body, maybe our personhood can be directed by the family relations around us, epigenetically modulated, like proteins, in unconscious ways. Maybe that is why this scene, more than countless others I had with doting grandparents on both sides of my family, is burned into my memory. "Just wait here, Brett, they'll come," he had whispered in the woods near Lincoln. "Who will come, Grandpa?" I want to shout now to this myth of a man, the one who smothered so much of my childhood in the dark drapes of Montana yearning. Was my CVID always coming, and was it always coming from him? Is the secret to my family history of illness hidden in the "family history" part of this deceptively simple question?

Charles Janeway was less clear on the acquired variety of CVID, but the congenital version of CVID originated from the maternal side of the family. In 1957, Gitlin and Janeway had written, "Many of the families' brothers or maternal uncles of the patients had died of what appeared to be agammaglobulinemia." They continued: "It is now clear that agammaglobulinemia is a hereditary disorder." Whether the acquired form, "like diabetes, is inherited as a tendency which manifests itself only later in life," triggered by environmental causes or even stress, remained a mystery to them, but the predisposition for the disease is certainly inherited.

CHAPTER 5

Phenotypes

L OOKING BACK INTO MY FAMILY'S HISTORY IS THE FINAL piece to this medical narrative, but one complicated by the fact that the cause of death for somebody who lived centuries ago is often nearly impossible to discern when few historical documents survive, let alone medical ones. Members of my family are mainly meat packers, coal miners, farmers, carpenters, day laborers, and small business owners, and they left precious little behind in the way of documentation. This sort of historical morbidity and mortality exploration also assumes that bacterial and viral infections have remained relatively unchanged over time, which is untrue: the body's microorganisms have evolved in historical time, altering the basic microbial composition of the human ecosystem. My body has a variety of bugs unique to my American, protein-rich diet, for example. I also live among tough bugs that have evolved to survive the era of antibiotic therapy. And it is untrue that my body has the same chemical composition as the bodies of my ancestors. Simply put, my body is an artifact of our industrial age; and my CVID might be, too.

According to the US Centers for Disease Control and Prevention (CDC), my body probably carries over two hundred environmental chemicals and their shifty metabolites, including disinfectants, environmental phenols, fungicides, herbicides, insecticides, metals, cosmetic preservatives, perchlorate and other anions, organofluorine compounds, phthalates and phthalate alternatives, phytoestrogens, polycyclic aromatic hydrocarbons, and volatile organic compounds. It is entirely possible that my CVID is the product of organic and synthetic chemicals such as these, as toxicologists have linked immunological diseases to such pollutants. It is possible that my ancestors had the genotype (genetic constitution of an individual) to express CVID—as my grandfather did to acquire diabetes—but just needed the right chemical trigger and, therefore, the right moment in history, when that chemical was present in the environment. I might have been at the wrong place, with the genetic potentiality, at the wrong historical time. Essentially, this is epigenetics, which are heritable changes to gene expression that occur without altering DNA sequences. In this manner, the investigation of my family's history is more than a search for evidence of heredity: it is also about historical contexts, such as environments, lifestyles, and occupations, because it is in contexts like these where epigenetic expressions and blockages can be triggered.

Environmental pollutants, for example, ranging from heavy metals to chemicals, can change genetic expression and trigger disease through such processes as DNA methylation (a epigenetic tool that can repress or block genetic transcription), histone modifications (posttranslational modification that influences gene expression and includes methylation), and microRNA expression (part of posttranscriptional genetic expression). I return to these, particularly histone modifications, in the epilogue. I happen to live in the age of disinfectants and plastics, for example, so I developed CVID as a result of their having permeated my porous body and blocked genetic expression within my white blood cells, while my ancestors with a similar genotype lived in a disinfectant-free and plastic-free age and did not develop CVID. This is precisely how my doctors talk about my CVID: I have the white blood cells, I have mature B-cells, for example, but something is blocking their secretion of antibodies in response to antigens. In sum, I am as much a phenotype (a collection of individual characteristics resulting from the interaction of genotypes and the environment) as I am a genotype, and when I think of the environment that shapes phenotypes—particularly diseased ones like me—I understand it to be a historically constructed context, something that changes throughout time and is the product of human decisions.

Importantly, history also connects to our earlier discussion of the biological formation of memory, because history represents disciplined, shared memories, an institutionalized appendage to our B-cells and neuronal forests. When reflecting on the importance of memory, Eric Kandel, the Nobel Prize–winning neurologist, wrote that remembering things is important not just for how people understand themselves but also for how societies understand themselves. "Memory is essential not only for the continuity of individual identity," he explained, "but also for the transmission of culture and for the evolution and continuity of societies over centuries." Memory, and history as a form of disciplined memory, is a key ingredient to the success of societies in this regard. We transmit our shared stories through history to generations of present and future citizens, and these become the shared stories that hold national communities together.

The principal difference between family history and histories of other forms of human organization, such as nations, is that most societies are cultural constructs that people forge over time through political imagination; so the continual rehearsal of a shared history, in order to understand the present and plot a future direction, is instrumental in maintaining cohesion. Really, there is nothing natural about a nation. By contrast, family history contains Ivan Doig's "blood words," ones that naturally link the present to the past in a concrete fashion, within the milieu of our plasma. Social cohesion in a multiethnic, multireligious, and multiclass society such as the United States does not naturally spring from the soil but, rather, is fashioned and learned through the political labor of people, and through the researching, writing, debating, and revising of the meaning of that society's history. My family history is more natural, built as it is from shared blood and certain genotypes; but it does not spring from the soil, either. It, too, has to be researched and written: it is not inscribed in my X-chromosome, for example.

But histories of societies are just as important as family histories, because societies have only history to knit them together. Societies that fail to transmit shared memory through history are doomed to grope through life as an Alzheimer's patient does, lost in a sea of unannounced encounters, unfamiliar faces, and in a frighteningly uncontextualized world. Consequently, a political mission of progress has driven the discipline of history from its nineteenth-century inception, as exemplified by such historians as Leopold von Ranke. Today, many historians pursue this political mission through gritty historical revisionism, such as in the case of social historians, where past injustices are brought to light for the purpose of promoting social equity. But less popular among academics is the idea that historians must also pursue the political mission of social cohesion by doing the ideological work of the nation, by reflecting on not just past injustices but also those unifying experiences that comprise a nation's past. It is important that historians identify the values that unite us, as well as those that divide us.

In these endeavors, the historical archive, such as the National Archives in Washington, DC, serves as a cultural appendage of the body's memory, and historians labor much as proteins do, building the long-term synaptic connections of social remembrance. Simply, they connect where we are today with how we got here. The boxes, files, shelves, and drawers that comprise the National Archive are not dissimilar to the biological architecture of Santiago Ramón y Cajal's neuronal forests: they, too, are epigenetic, as historians build them from the life experiences that made a sensory impression on us all, and which are passed down to future generations. And history modulates society much as a mother's B-cells and antibodies modulate a baby's immune system. The human brain may be good at building protein-created synaptic connections for long-term memory storage, but the brain rots, like everything else related to "the material me" does, when we die. History, as the contentious enterprise of preserving and interrogating memories and stories, represents the social transcendence of the finitude of the organ we call the brain. History serves as the long-term repository of shared stories, one that we debate and dispute, but ultimately, pass down to others for the continuing project of building cohesion in our communities. The historical archive, then, is the cultural elaboration of the immune system and neuronal architecture, and as such it is critical to our development and defense as a social species.

My comparison of the historical archive to neuronal forests, and the historian to a memory-creating protein, is not just some pointy-headed meditation on biological determinism and scientific reductionism, hallmarks of the entire Enlightenment project that dominates modern science, and which is often more distracting than useful in the humanities. In fact, by identifying the role of thousands of microorganisms in creating our individual person, I am doing the opposite of reducing. But reductionism is a powerful part of post-Enlightenment thought, and history, as an academic discipline, was born from the same primordial Enlightenment stew as other academic disciplines, particularly those in the sciences. The early-seventeenth-century father of investigative science, Francis Bacon, dispelled magic and mystery in nature and the body in favor of an intrusive experimental science. He sought to discover the basic elements that made us function, as well as the mechanistic patterns and particulars that he believed governed the universe. Joseph Glanvill elaborated on Bacon's project when he argued that the purpose of science is to "enlarge knowledge by observation and experiment . . . so that nature being known, it may be mastered, managed, and used in the services of human life." Once the scientist "eviscerates" nature, Glanvill wrote, this leads to the "disclosure of the springs of its motion," or its internal mechanisms. Glanvill understood the importance of scale, and that the microscope is critical to this reductionist enterprise because "the secrets of nature are not in the greater masses, but in those little threads and springs which are too subtle for the grossness of our unhelped senses." As with Janeway's blood fractions or Cajal's neurons, the microscope allowed the scientist to transcend the "grossness of our unhelped senses" to see those "little threads and springs" that together comprise the patterns of the body and the physical universe.

The Enlightenment crafted a machinelike image of the body and society, one built from smaller parts that could, with the help of microscopy and other techniques and technologies, be disassembled to reveal how things worked, and then reassembled in order to control them and, finally, market them for the betterment of bourgeois life. This mechanical and quantifiable reductionism served as the principle of the philosophies of René Descartes and Thomas Hobbes as well, both of whom carried the Enlightenment's mantle after Bacon and Glanvill. "No qualities are known which are so occult and no effects of sympathy and antipathy so marvelous and strange, and finally nothing else in nature so rare . . . for which the reason cannot be given by means of the same principles," insisted Descartes. Disassemble the living machine of the body, and its basic mathematical principles, the laws of its motion, its material particles, and those "little threads and springs" that make it function can be exposed, identified, controlled, and, in my case, replaced when they are absent.

I am alive because of the Enlightenment's approach to medicine: reduce it to see what is there and, in my case, what is missing or broken, and then fix it, not unlike repairing an old Ford pickup. These patterns could be expanded and this basic reductionism transferred to theories of social cohesion as well. "God set up mathematical laws in nature as a king sets up laws in his kingdom," Descartes wrote in 1630. Just like the human body described by Descartes, individual people became the particulars of the social body, the ordering of which was Hobbes's principal interest. Society was a machine for Hobbes, much like the body. "For what is the heart," he pondered, "but a spring; and the nerves, but so many springs; and the joints, but so many wheels, giving motion to the whole body, such as was intended by the artificer?" For Enlightenment thinkers, the body and society as a whole became machines that could be tinkered with, disassembled, and thereby understood.

What I mean by not being a reductionist is that I view the body as more ecosystem-like than isolated, as more porous than contained behind an epidermal wall, and I view history as governed more by patterns, structures, and contexts than by the will of individuals; mine is not a mission of reducing and simplify-ing but of introducing the complexity of even more voices—the voices of the microbiotic world of the immunologically com-promised body. What Janeway witnessed when he looked under his microscope was not only the isolated bands of albumin and immunoglobulins but also the increasing complexities of molec-ular, cellular, and even viral and bacteriological communities within the individual person's body. The closer he looked, the more complex and interconnected the picture became. Though Hobbes viewed people as cells in the body politic, Janeway and others discovered that the body itself constituted a community, one composed of bacteria with which we are in constant bidirec-tional communication. A CVID patient such as myself is also in constant battle with them, even fairly benign ones. Importantly, the microbiologist's broadening of the parameters of what con-stitutes "the material me" parallels the historian's broadening of parameters involved in constructing the social us—the closer you look, the more thoroughly you investigate; and the more you shape the theoretical lens, the more complex society gets and the more voices historians are required to include. If indi-vidual men once drove history as the autonomous human body once drove medicine, then history is now seen as driven by com-plex communities of people, not unlike the complex microbial communities that direct our bodies through life in a story of bio-logical mutualism. It is the seemingly endless patterns of com-plexity that make things work in this world, not their reduced simplicity. Just because I use medicine and biology in this book, and talk of genotypes and phenotypes, for example, does not automatically mean that I am a determinist or a reductionist—I am quite the opposite, in fact.

This is what I have learned in my family history of illness so far: I have learned to reject the notion of the primacy of

the autonomous self in history and have discovered the importance of looking beyond the Edifice-of-Me to understand what
I am. The imagined me is a decider, a transcendent being independently guiding my way through life with agency and willful
choices. "The material me," by contrast, is a product of biological and historical codependencies, coevolutions, genetic and
phenotypic development, and thick layers of context, a being
who cannot be understood outside his life's biological and
historical milieu. I have come to privilege the overwhelming
material context of my life into which I have been thrown and
through which I navigate, because, as a phenotype, I was partly
made by my environment. As much as I have shaped my life
with my bare hands, my life direction is also about thick layers
of context: genetic context, epigenetic context, environmental
context, family context, and historical context. It is upon this
material reality that I sail, not as some isolated boat ghosting
through the glassy waters of a formless and historyless world.
It is always less about the boat than about the water and wind.

— · —

I first discovered the power of historical context in understanding the world when I took a Western Civilization course at the
College of Idaho, a wonderful liberal arts college that changed
my life in numerous ways. The persistent obsession with Montana farm life, the one that had drowned out everything else
in my cognitive world, including schoolwork, faded abruptly
as primitive visions of historical patterns consumed my newly
awoken academic imagination. For the first time in my life, I
actually became a student. History, more than any other field,
explained the world. I had told my parents that I did not want
to go to college after graduating from high school, but I reluctantly agreed to give it a try for a semester. I do not think I called

them until Thanksgiving, several months later. I became consumed by my new academic passion and Idaho's drinking age of
nineteen. I enrolled in a wide spectrum of courses in my major
and studied everything from classical and Asian history to US
intellectual history and the Holocaust. I also became intensely
interested in geology, in large part because it analyzed change
across time and explained why the physical word around me
looked the way that it did. The analysis of change over time just
resonated with me. I quit the ski team after realizing my skills
were grossly inadequate compared to those of the fast Cana-
dian racers on my team, and I began focusing on my studies.
It was slow going, as I had twelve years of academic disinterest
and lackluster performance to overcome, particularly in my
abysmal writing. In higher education, there is much discussion
about what entices students into successful learning. For me,
the recipe was simple, and I suspect that despite the millions we
spend on the "student services" industry in higher education,
it still is: the talent and charisma of my superb teachers was
irreplaceable (and I have never forgotten that golden rule in my
own approach to the classroom).

Obviously, when I walked into that Western Civilization
class in 1985, I had no idea of the momentous shifts that the
discipline of history had undergone in the preceding decade.
In some respects, historians had started to reject grand constructed patterns for deconstructed microhistories, because
they viewed the world's pattern constructors as biased people in
positions of patriarchal, capitalist, sectarian, or kinship-based
power. These patterns were no longer natural, moreover:
they were fabricated, invented out of thin air, to legitimize
that power. I started the study of history when the discipline
was in the throes of what would become known as historical
deconstructionism, the dismantling of the framework of past

historical models in favor of the "linguistic turn," or "cultural turn." If the nineteenth-century father of the academic discipline of history, Ranke, had urged historians to show the past "as it really had been," positioning the historian as a narrator more than as an analyzer of the past, then the field I walked into was highly analytic, with less empirical description, because critics viewed narrative itself as just another cultural invention. Ranke's self-proclaimed "archival curiosity" drove his obsession for empiricism, which placed him in the Enlightenment tradition of Bacon and others in crafting a God's-eye view of events. Events were out there, suspended in archival amber, and the historian just had to go out and find them. Ranke submitted that a "return to the most pristine sources," those drafted by eyewitnesses to key historical events, fostered the "rise of pure perception" in the historian's mind. The importance of the historian's "pure perception" was simple: "History has been assigned to the office of judging the past and of instructing the present for the benefit of future ages," he optimistically explained. Historians are like social proteins.

Despite his nineteenth-century appeal to historians, that they describe the past as "it really had been," Ranke was anything but apolitical in his approach to the past. Such towering men as Martin Luther and Frederick II drove Ranke's dramatic and often triumphant narratives, and his obsession with written primary sources inexorably led him away from the powerless masses of illiterates that comprised the bulk of his world. After the publication of his history of Prussia, he admitted as much when he remarked, "I do not deny that I display a lively sympathy with the events I describe—the rise of the state— but without such sympathy a book of this kind could not have been written." He, too, was interested in patterns in the past, the patterns within which states and international relations resided. "Nature itself strives to produce form," he argued, "and the works of the mind must strive in the same direction." In some respects, nature's form is one of the keys to understanding Ranke's organization of the past, but Ranke remained so focused on the political elite that it was almost inevitable that historians armed with a broader social approach would radically redirect the study of the past. Ranke was not necessarily leaving out the voices of common people intentionally. He was searching for structure, some kind of theoretical scaffolding on which to build his narrative, and the "rise of the state" and the "genius" of Prussian princes provided that structure. These Prussian princes were the thinking agents of history. Only when a new structure found its voice, a Marxist structure of material production in history, did historians begin to depart from the story of states and princes and chart a new course in describing and analyzing the past in the framework of production, class development, and political struggle.

Being confined to the political elite, Ranke's approach to the past is not helpful for the present investigation of my family history of illness, because most of my family, with a few exceptions, were the lower sort that remained largely outside traditional historical narratives. There are no historical archives filled with their official documents that would have opened a window into their inner political musings; rather, there are only traces of my family in ships' manifests, federal censuses, marriage licenses, vital records, and other colorless asides. It is impossible for the historian to enter their minds to determine the reasoning behind their choices, or even their possible sicknesses and causes of death. But they are part of a class of people who, through their collective labor and production, undeniably drove history, so social history brings us closer to a theoretical structure that can elucidate my family's history.

Social historians drew on Marxist theories of history because production and class development broadened the parameters regarding who participated in history. The material economic conditions of individuals, more than what they thought, made them who they were. "As individuals express their life, so they are," wrote Karl Marx. "What they are, therefore, coincides with what they produce, with *what* they produce and *how* they produce. The nature of individuals thus depends on the material conditions which determine their production." This productive life, in turn, drove conscious life. Marx explained that "consciousness does not determine life, but life determines consciousness." In other words, Ranke's Prussian princes thought the way they did because they were princes, not vice versa. Marx took direct aim at empiricists such as Ranke when he wrote, "When this active life process is presented, history ceases to be a collection of dead facts as it is with the empiricists." Under this definition, the fact that my family members had existed within certain material conditions of production, as farmers, meat packers, and miners, meant they had a history. "History is nothing but the succession of separate generations," Marx wrote, "each of which exploits the material, capital, and productive forces handed down to it by all preceding generations." Much as I have in my family history of illness, Marx privileged the material milieu of our world when he mused, "Circumstances make men just as men make circumstances." He then elaborated: "Men make their own history, but they do not make it just as they please; they do not make it under circumstances chosen by themselves, but under circumstances directly encountered, given and transmitted from the past." He concluded: "The tradition of all the dead generations weighs like a nightmare on the brain of the living." The same is true of the social, biological, and genetic milieu that I was thrown into. Significantly, Marx anticipated Martin Heidegger and Charles Sherrington in ways that are important to my family history of illness.

Production and class became the principal concern of pioneering social historians such as Edward P. Thompson. How could you even approach a family's history without taking into account Marx's "*what* they produce and *how* they produce," the productive dimensions of their life experiences? As Thompson asked, "How is it possible to get very far with the discussion of household or family if we don't know whether the households were of serfs or freemen, fishermen or bakers, nomadic shepherds or miners, were cultivating rice or silk or chestnuts, what kind of inheritance customs determined the transmission of land, what kind of dowries or marriage settlements, what customs of apprenticeship or migrant labor?" He sought to rescue these people from the "enormous condescension of posterity," or Ranke's elitist approach, and place them front and center in British social existence. England's working class, he insisted, "was present at its own making," allotting the poor a voice in history where they seldom had one. Importantly, historians perceived class development as a common pattern in historical progress, and so it was easily exported to the study of societies other than industrial Europe: it was represented as a structure that promised to unify the seemingly divergent currents of world history. No matter the country, everybody is engaged in some sort of production and, eventually, class struggle.

My early family history holds together more by sinews of labor than it does by princely ponderings, though I do have ancestors who served as "freemen" in the General Court at Plymouth in the seventeenth century. What mostly drove my family's movement through history and across the continent from Plymouth to Great Falls was "*what* they produce and *how* they produce," or business or labor opportunities. I can trace my father's family to early US colonial settlement in Massachusetts. Originally, the Walker family started in England, in small villages and towns largely clustered south and southwest of London, but some were from towns in the north, around Manchester, as well. The Anglo-Saxon surname *Walker* is closely tied to Marx's *"what* they produce and *how* they produce," as the name is an alternative term for "fuller," or somebody who walked on woolen cloth in order to rid it of impurities and enlarge it. Presumably, my earliest English ancestors were fullers, involved in what the Welch still describe as "waulking" on cloth in water mills scattered across England, though there is a Sir William Walker (1399–1424) from Clapham Common. There is no record of his being knighted, so I assume he was a baronet, as the title became popular in the fourteenth century. William Walker III (1620–1703) made the journey to the New World sometime between 1620 and 1654, where he married Sarah Snow in Eastham, a newly created town on Cape Cod.

In 1640, a handful of Plymouth settlers, including Governor William Bradford, had set out for the "territory of the Nausets" to open up new farmlands and fishing grounds because of the cramped quarters and lousy soil at Plymouth. Settlers had known of Nauset territory since 1620, when they had first explored Cape Cod. In April 1644, seven Plymouth colonists and their families, some forty-nine people in all, settled on lands they purchased from local Indians, which amounted to the towns of Orleans, Eastham, and Wellfleet. In June 1646, the General Court in Plymouth granted Nauset "to be a township, and to have all the privileges of a township as other towns within the government have," and the founders elected officers the next year. In 1651, the General Court ordered that the "town of Nauset be henceforth called and known as Eastham," erasing the town's Indian origins, and the entire territory became Eastham until Wellfleet and Orleans separated in the eighteenth century. Without delay, the settlers cultivated their "plantation" of wheat, corn, beans, and other crops while also exploiting fisheries, digging shellfish, and producing salt in the surrounding tidal lands. Relations between Eastham settlers and nearby Native Americans remained tense and unsettled until most land claims were resolved in 1666. By 1695, residents had "built the stocks and whipping post near the church," and consequently, the stern rhythms of New England civil life had begun.

William more or less kept his nose clean, at least according to General Court Treasury Accounts from Plymouth. He avoided fines for "being drunke" and "carnall coppulation," but he did pick up a small fine in June 1671 for "telling a lye." Sadly, the treasury offered no specific information about the nature of his fib, but the Puritan scrutiny probably proved stifling. "Telling a lye" did not disqualify William from joining the ranks of New England's governing freemen, and in 1658 and 1689 he took the "Oath of Fidelitie" for Eastham. Later, in 1695, William and his two sons, William Jr. and Jabez, are listed as among freemen, which meant that the entire Walker family qualified by belonging to the Plymouth church and by owning a notable "estate." Until 1660, such freemen served as legislators who traveled to Plymouth to cast votes at the General Court, while after that they often voted by proxy. William probably became a fixture in Eastham before he died in 1703 at the ripe old age of eighty-three, so surely he, having withstood the scrutiny of Puritan mores and the death-grip of seventeenth-century epidemiological mayhem, was not the hereditary harbinger of my CVID. If not William, then who?

With CVID, what we are looking for is a rare disease, affecting one person per fifty thousand to two hundred thousand people, depending on the context. Although Janeway believed CVID to be mostly inherited, recent medical research suggests that the acquired variety of CVID is probably as much a sporadic disease as a hereditary one, with maybe as few as 20 percent of cases being the result of family inheritance, typically the autosomal-dominant variety. Briefly, *autosomal* means that the gene in question is a non-sex chromosome, while *dominant* means that a single copy of the genetic mutation is enough to cause the disease. Physicians have observed patients ranging in age from three to seventy-nine, but the onset of symptoms usually occurs at twenty-three years for men and twenty-eight years for women. Usually, diagnosis occurs at twenty-nine and thirty-three years, respectively. Simply put, my search for the hereditary origins of my CVID is like searching for an autosomal-inheritance needle in a historical haystack, but the first place to start is with life expectancies and causes of mortality in seventeenth-century colonial America. I need a baseline with which to compare the lifespans of my New England ancestors.

Life expectancies for men in seventeenth-century Europe hovered at about sixty-seven years, plus or minus nine years, if one lived to see his twentieth birthday; the life expectancy for women proved considerably lower, at fifty-seven years. This means that a twenty-year-old man living in England in 1650, for example, might be expected to live, on average, between fifty-eight and seventy-six years, while his wife likely occupied the low end of that spectrum. In seventeenth-century Plymouth Colony, near Eastham, where William and his wife, Sarah, settled in 1654, colonists who lived to see their twentieth birth-days had an average life expectancy of just under seventy years. This is because most seventeenth-century endemic diseases winnowed out children and young people, who were still in the process of developing acquired immunities to bacterial and viral infections. Infants and small children born with immunological challenges such as CVID or Bruton's syndrome would have died well before reaching twenty. Settlers faced an onslaught of dangerous endemic and epidemic diseases, including typhus, dysentery, smallpox, influenza, whooping cough, diphtheria, scarlet fever, yellow fever, and measles. These contagions determined when people lived, when they became ill, and when they died. William, my earliest New England ancestor, and his son Jabez both exceeded the average life expectancy in colonial America. Their wives, Sarah and Elizabeth, also met or exceeded the average life expectancy.

However, Jabez and Elizabeth's son, Jeremiah, died young, at thirty-eight, which immediately attracted my attention. Since nearly all colonial vital records do not list a cause of death, it is next to impossible to determine precisely what killed him, and the Massachusetts Historical Society archives, which I searched, also lack this information. But once he had turned thirty years old, he was statistically expected to live until he was over seventy, so something cut Jeremiah's life short, even after he had presumably been exposed to an onslaught of bacterial and viral endemic contagions that killed other colonists in droves. Furthermore, his wife, Esther, lived for nearly a century, making Jeremiah's death even more a mystery. Something killed him, and him alone. If, for example, an epidemic ravaged Eastham, Needham, or Harwich, why did Esther survive and Jeremiah perish? Did his body, at the age of thirty-eight years, simply stop producing antibodies, as mine did in Minneapolis, and make him vulnerable to infection and death? It is possible that disease killed him, because in the colonies smallpox increased in virulence between about 1730 and 1760, and "scattered outbreaks of measles" hit New England between 1739 and 1741. In the case of measles, for example, evidence exists that as people fled Boston they carried the infection with them, and some may have fled to Harwich. Smallpox and measles are both viruses that kill people even under the best immunological circumstances, but that raises the question why Esther survived. Jeremiah's death sticks out as a possible example of the hereditary predisposition for CVID; but with Janeway's medical research into blood fractions over two centuries down the road, it is impossible to know for sure. What I would not do for a small vial of his blood.

Jeremiah may have died young, but his son, Benjamin, lived to see his ninetieth year, as did Benjamin's wife, Sylvia. However, Benjamin's death in 1816 strangely corresponds with the deaths of his son and daughter-in-law: Marshall Walker and his wife, Hannah, died within a week of each other in 1816, in their midfifties, which attracted my attention as well, but for reasons other than Jeremiah's early death. I suspect their deaths related to the infamous "year without a summer," which resulted from climatological shifts caused by the volcanic eruption of Mount Tambora on the Indonesian island of Sumbawa. In April 1815, Mount Tambora erupted in one of the largest volcanic blasts in history. The explosion spread a sulfate aerosol veil across much of North America, including the colonies, in the spring and summer of 1815, which decreased air temperatures and caused a series of food shortages. "The sun, ere he sank among the dark western clouds, shot out," wrote one observer from the British Isles, "a light so angry, yet so ghastly, that it gave the whole earth a wild, alarming and spectral hue, like that seen in some feverish dream." It was in this climate of a "feverish dream" that Mary Shelley told the story of Frankenstein's monster while with inspired friends in Switzerland.

In Ireland a different monster irrupted, the disease typhus, which thrived with the cold temperatures and food shortages, infecting a third of the inhabitants of Dublin and killing thousands. One writer recalled that with the typhus epidemic, the "gloom that darkened the face of the country had become awful. . . . Typhus fever had now set in, and was filling the land with fearful and unexampled desolation. Famine, in all cases the source and origin of contagion, had done, and was still doing, its work." The reasons for the typhus outbreak relate not only to the malnutrition caused by the "year without a summer" but also to people spending more time indoors, sharing clothing more often, huddling together, and cleaning their linens and clothing less, allowing lice to proliferate. The bacterium that causes epidemic typhus, *Rickettsia prowazekii*, inhabits lice feces, and it spread easily in the relentlessly cold temperatures and damp weather that followed the eruption. The bacterium infects lice bite wounds. It then multiplies in the blood stream and damages the gastrointestinal tract and other vital organs at a cellular level. Starting out as confused and feverish, one in four victims eventually dies from painful organ failure.

With the exception of Jeremiah, then, most Walkers lived out their full life expectancy, some of them far exceeding their life expectancy. Even when they did not, as in the case of Marshall and Hannah, I can use epidemiological history to contextualize their deaths in a manner that provides plausible explanations for their dying relatively young. The "year without a summer" and its accompanying diseases affected New England in a manner that would explain why Marshall and Hannah died in their fifties and within a week of each other. Coincidence is not a satisfactory explanation for their deaths. They might have been trying to just keep warm in the persistent damp and colder-than-normal temperatures, huddled together in their humble home with the elderly Benjamin, but in doing so they exposed themselves to lice and their parasitic bacteria. They ultimately contracted typhus, and it killed them. No such historical explanation remains for Jeremiah, however, and I am left to wonder what caused him to die in his thirties. But if Jeremiah did have a hereditary predisposition for CVID, or something like it, presumably it would emerge elsewhere in the Walker line, as the genetic potentiality would continue to get passed down in the family's blood.

— · —

Not unlike the blizzard I watched from my hospital bed in Minneapolis, where the conical, white beam of light provided by a streetlamp had briefly illuminated the snowflakes that passed underneath, the Walker family, too, largely disappeared into the darkness. They stopped orbiting the Plymouth colony and moved out from under the light of history that shown on the founding of the United States. Silently, my family began to wash across the continent, following the incoming tide of Indian genocide as Native Americans succumbed to European colonial settlement. Marshall Keith Walker and his wife, Anna Maria, pulled up their New England roots and relocated to Hamlin, Pennsylvania. In 1850, according to the 1850 US Census, Marshall and his family lived in Gibson, almost due north of Scranton. In June 1863, during the Civil War, he registered for military duty in Pennsylvania's Eleventh Congressional District but, to my knowledge, never saw combat. On the fertile soil of Pennsylvania, Marshall Keith and Anna Maria had twelve children, including their son Nelson Lemuel Walker. Nelson and his wife, Polly Ann, had two sons, one of them, Neal Victor Walker, was my great-grandfather. But between Neal Victor and me stretches one of the most formidable historical chasms in the researching and writing of this book. Neal Victor is an enigma in my genealogical time line, one that requires a radical retooling of my theoretical lens. Up to this point, a Marxist lens of *what* they produce and *how* they produce" has served our purposes, largely explaining the Walker family's humble textile-industry beginning and their "estate" in Eastham, which qualified William and his two boys to serve as freemen in the Plymouth General Court. Other than the information about William's fine for "telling a lye," I know the New England Walkers only by their social class, by their belonging to the Plymouth church, not by their individual actions. But a Marxist focus on production can explain only part of Neal Victor's choices. My grandfather, father, and I were never

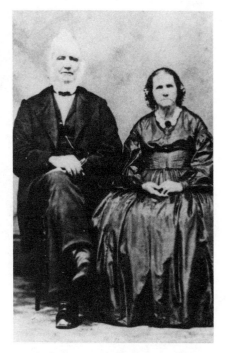

Marshall Keith and Anna Maria Walker, my great-great-great-grandparents

connected to Neal Victor through personal relationships or even stories—neither my grandfather nor my father ever met him—but we were connected to him by blood, which makes him an important link in my genealogical chain and my family history of illness.

Neal Victor was born to Nelson and Polly Ann on January 13, 1874, in Nicholson, Pennsylvania. He attended Princeton University as a member of the class of 1895 but never graduated from the Ivy League institution. In 1896, he married and briefly moved to Buffalo, New York, for employment. However, in July 1897 he returned to the Nicholson area, where he planned to help manage a lumber business owned by his father.

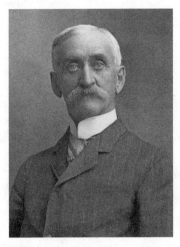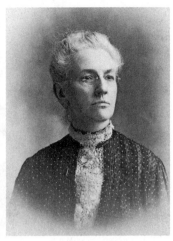

Nelson Walker, my great-great-grandfather, and Polly Ann Walker, my great-great-grandmother

But business affairs went poorly for Neal Victor, and in June 1900, in front of the Scranton City Court House, his property in Highland Park went up for auction because of unpaid taxes. Within months, he had moved with his wife, Mary, to South Abington, Pennsylvania, and in 1906 he attended an event at the Elm Park United Methodist Church in Scranton, where he worked as a freight agent. Four years later, however, he and Mary had moved to Aurora, Missouri, where they had (or possibly adopted) a daughter named Elizabeth. In September 1918, his World War I draft card listed his occupation as that of city commissioner. The family of three lived together in Aurora in 1920. By 1930, however, Neal Victor was divorced and living alone. In that intervening decade, something important, if not more than a little scandalous, occurred in my family's history.

My paternal grandfather, Neal Lawrence Walker, whom I knew well, was born to Neal Victor and Bonnie Louise Schnur, my great-grandmother known as Louise, whom I also remember quite well. Neal Victor, it seems, had had an affair with a woman thirty years younger than him, which led to the dissolution of his marriage and his living alone for the rest of his life as a lodger. He died that way: alone and paralyzed in Kansas City, struck down by arteriosclerosis and heart disease. According to Neal Victor's Standard Certificate of Death, his father was "unknown," his mother was "unknown," and he had "no relatives," and that was the way he remained until I started researching this book. His body had been donated to scientific research, probably sliced open by giggling undergraduates somewhere. It turns out, however, that he did have relatives— and I am one of them. It is a jarring chasm in an American family genealogy that extends to the original Plymouth Colony. When I started writing this book, my father asked me if I knew anything about Neal Victor, his grandfather, and the Walker family beyond my dad's father. My father, and his father, had never met the man. My grandfather, after graduating from high school, had traveled to Missouri to find his dad, only to be told that he had "just missed him." He had died two years earlier. "You're too late, young man," my grandfather was told at the lodge. My purpose in this project was never to uncover the fact that my grandfather was a bastard, but that is precisely what happened. "That's a hell of a secret for a family to keep," my father said when I finally explained Neal Victor's story to him.

With Neal Victor, though, ideas, possibly powerfully big-oted ideas, replaced Marxist notions of production in driving his life choices. Unpaid Pennsylvania taxes could have been what prompted Neal Victor's move to Aurora, where in 1910 he earned a wage as superintendent of a water company, but other work, a particular kind of ideological work, might better explain his deci-sion to move to Aurora. Think about it: he came from a Plym-outh colonial family that had never been south of Scranton, and he suddenly decided to move to Aurora, Missouri, to be a water company superintendent? I doubt it. In 1920, Neal Victor worked as a "manager" in a "publishing house," and the largest publishing house in Aurora in 1920 was that of a newspaper titled *The Menace*, a virulently anti-Catholic rag with a large distribution. (My grandfather had always told my father that Neal Victor was a "newspaper man.") The newspaper appealed to "patriotic men," some of them with possible family connections to Plymouth Colony, and served as a "machine for fighting for the liberties of the American people." Serving as a water company superintendent might not explain the move to Aurora, but "fighting for the liberties of the American people" just might. *The Menace* was launched in an old Aurora opera house in 1911, when the city's population was just over four thousand. By 1915, the newspaper had about 1.5 million subscribers nationwide and dwarfed the more famous newspapers of Chicago and New York. It defined life in Aurora at this time, and many people in the town were involved with the newspaper in one capacity or another. In September 1914, the Menace Publishing Company was incorporated as the United States Publishing Company, and it made stock options available to "patriotic citizens of the United States whose loyalty to the principles for which we stand is unquestioned." *The Menace* identified Aurora as "the World's Headquarters for Anti-Papal Literature," and in 1916, after the newspaper won a federal obscenity case, the defendants, as they returned from court, were met in Aurora by "an immense crowd comprising more than half the population gathered at the depot." This crowd was, as one observer explained, "headed by [a] band, and when the defendants stepped from the train they were royally welcomed." According to one account, the Aurora Post Office tripled its workers to handle the massive distributional requirements. The newspaper railed against state governments "dominated by

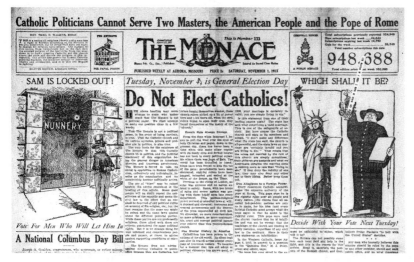

The anti-Catholic *Menace* newspaper, published in Aurora, Missouri, between 1911 and 1920

Roman catholic 'drunks'" and threatened to spark a patriotic national revolution. "If we are compelled to live in this country with Romanists, as our weak-kneed Protestant critics say we are, the Romanists will have to be taught their place in society," the newspaper snarled to its xenophobic readers.

It could be that one thread that tugged at Neal Victor's conscience was his patriotic Plymouth roots—his ties to freeman William and his wife, Sarah Snow—as well as xenophobic fears of the Roman Catholic papal scourge so viciously portrayed in *The Menace*. Patriotism is an idea, a very powerful idea, one that fills the pages of the anti-Catholic newspaper, and such ideas often motivate people to do things outside their simple economic best interest, thereby undermining many Marxist and rational-choice interpretations of history. Could it be that Neal Victor first subscribed to *The Menace* while in Pennsylvania and then decided to move to Aurora to be on "the Firing Line," as the

newspaper frequently characterized its Aurora writers and workers? Was living in the "World's Headquarters for Anti-Papal Literature" appealing to him? In many respects, this kind of example,
of historical actors being motivated by things other than their
economic best interests, sparked the 1980s cultural turn in history because it better explained what really motivated people,
such as blue-collar workers voting in droves to elect as president
Ronald W. Reagan, whose "trickle down" economic policies
mainly benefited wealthier folks. When I attended graduate
school at Portland State University and the University of Oregon
in the 1990s, the cultural turn had a firm grip on most academic
historians and defined the direction of the field because it promised to explain the place of identity, such as being a Protestant
American patriot, in history. As a graduate student, I was trained
under the heavy influence of the cultural turn.

— . —

The cultural turn started in the late 1970s, when historians such
as Raymond Williams began emphasizing the importance of
culture in determining historical events and choices. He still
worked within the Marxist framework of historical materialism,
but culture came to hold increased explanatory value. Williams
never viewed culture as distinct from material life but instead
saw it as operating within webs of social relationships and material objects. Critical cultural phenomena, such as language, religion, nationalism, and other ideological production, occurred
as "indissoluble elements of the material social process itself,
involved all the time both in production and reproduction."
For Williams, Marx's focus on "*what* they produce and *how*
they produce" also applied to cultural production, which he
viewed as driving historical change. But Williams served only
as a transitional figure between social history and the cultural

turn, and a new generation of historians became increasingly dissatisfied with the requirement to tether historical interpretation to material life. Language and culture became historical drivers that transcended material life through creating forms of identity, such as Neal Victor's possible desire to be included among "patriotic men." The cultural turn dissected history and extracted culture from its productive, institutional, and historical contexts and unleashed it as a powerful explanatory phantasm, one that created a whole new constellation of categories of analysis, such as gender, race, and ethnicity—people became more than the sum of their economic best-interested parts. In explaining Neal Victor's life, his labor as a freight agent probably means little, but his identity as a Protestant patriot with family ties to the Plymouth church probably meant a great deal to him. I never knew of these genealogical ties, because of the chasm of illegitimacy that separated my great-grandfather and me, but had I known of them, had they been taught to me by my father, they probably would have been important to me, too.

The cultural turn and its new retinue of categories proved inherently interdisciplinary, with a variety of cultural theoreticians redirecting history away from Marx's materialism. The cultural turn was principally about language and categories, all of them subject to the scrutiny of historical analysis. The literary critic Edward Said wrote, "All knowledge that is about human society . . . is historical knowledge, and therefore rests upon judgment and interpretation." Everything within human society, every word, every grammatical fragment, and every category, every assumption and conceit, and every ethical norm, was historically constructed and therefore subject to interpretation. "This is not to say that facts or data are nonexistent," he cautioned, "but that facts get their importance from what is made of them in interpretation." Said argued that interpretation itself was historically contingent, "for interpretations depend very much on who the interpreter is, who he or she is addressing, what his or her purpose is, at what historical moment the historical interpretation takes place." Every category became relational and relative under Said's formulation, every normative statement a historically contingent cultural relic of a past age. Similarly, Benedict Anderson, a scholar of Asia, argued that nations, one of the basic political features of modern life, represented one such category, and that rather than view nations as "facts," one had to view them as historical constructs. Anderson argued that nations are imagined, not something that naturally springs from the soil, because "members of even the smallest nation will never know most of their fellow-members, meet them, or even hear of them, yet in the mind of each lives the image of their communion." He presented the nation as entirely conjured from the political imagination, denying it any material existence that might transcend human subjectivity. This interrogation of the words and categories of history even deconstructed the basic narrative structure with which historians most often communicate.

Hayden White, a historian and literary critic, suggested that because the "narrative mode of representation" appears so natural to human communication, "its use in any field of study aspiring to the status of a science must be suspect." He wagged his finger at the entire discipline when he explained that the "continued use by historians of a narrative mode of representation is an index of a failure at once methodological and theoretical." He contended that a "discipline that produces narrative accounts of its subject matter as an end in itself seems methodologically unsound," because historical events do not unfold as tightly knit stories. In other words, telling stories, much as I am doing in this book, is a radical distortion of the past. White concluded that the "notion that sequences of real events possess the formal attributes of the stories we tell about imaginary events could only have its origin in wishes, daydreams, reveries." White reduced the historical classics to a fictional wasteland of empirically justified daydreams.

The interpretative dissection of vocabularies, grammars, categories of analysis, and narrative modes of representation mattered because, once historicized, they often exposed the "anonymous instruments of power" that created them and used them for the political purpose of wielding influence. In social history, the bourgeoisie exercised economic power over labor and production; but after the cultural turn, true power was exercised more subtly, in more symbolic realms, and in such institutions as hospitals, mental health institutions, social norms, and prisons. It was even exercised in common practices such as sexual relations. Such vocabularies and categories as "family," "history," and even "illness" all proved historically contingent and, thus, with the cultural turn, required interpretative unpacking—much as I'm doing in this book. With cultural turn historians, there was no God's-eye view of events, no vantage point of universal unbiased understanding, no disciplinary methodology that transcended the milieu of historical influence—everything, even the grandest hypothesis, was socially embedded, relative, and contingent. Few unpacked categories and institutions better than philosopher Michel Foucault, who expanded the interpretive archive of the historian in imaginative ways. Foucault's studies rejected the idea of "universal structures" and instead viewed all words and categories, even our most basic moral assumptions, as "many historical events." Foucault referred to the interrogation of words, practices, and categories as "archaeology" and "genealogy," which described the search for cognitive lineages with the past, and usually this investigation uncovered the association between ideas, discipline, and power.

The techniques of discipline were never solely about economics, either. Foucault conceded that "bio-power," the disciplining of bodies, included the "controlled insertion of bodies into the machinery of production," but this sort of capitalism was also about confining people, making bodies docile, punishing people, and institutionalizing them. "The perfect disciplinary apparatus would make it possible for a single gaze to see everything constantly," wrote Foucault, and for the controller of that increasingly creepy gaze to be the "perfect eye that nothing would escape." It is because of Foucault that Joan W. Scott, in her famous 1986 article on gender, started out by explaining, "Words, like the ideas and things they are meant to signify, have a history." History became less the study of events than the study of the analytical categories used to explain those events, including words. Not unlike a body with an autoimmune disorder, history turned against itself and began several decades' worth of self-interrogation and, in many instances, self-destruction as a result of the cultural turn. I do not mean to be overly critical, however, because the cultural turn shaped my approach to history. The cultural turn created a generation of historians masterful at re-creating historical identities, which helps us understand economically irrational choices, ones motivated by ideas such as patriotism. This is the idea that I suspect motivated Neal Victor Walker.

— · —

Louise, my great-grandmother, raised my grandfather Neal in Casper. She remarried several times. Neal eventually married my grandmother Dorothy Nelson, from Saint Paul, Minnesota. Dorothy's father was from River Falls, Wisconsin, but both of his parents, John O. Nelson and Mathilda Segerstrom, had immigrated to the United States from Skåne County on the

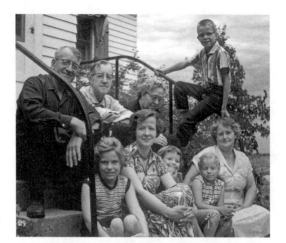

The Nelson family in North Dakota. My paternal grandmother, Dorothy, is seated in the middle; my father, Nelson, sits on the railing.

southernmost tip of Sweden. Mathilda died at forty-six, about the age I would have died had I not lived when I lived; and her mother, Johanna Kjertindotter, also died earlier than her life expectancy predicted. Mathilda's father, Nickolas Segerstrom, lived to see his eighty-fourth year. That Dorothy lived hard her whole life, drinking, playing bridge, and smoking cigarettes, and still managed to live to seventy-five years of age, appears to disqualify the Swedish branch of my family as the potential source of my hereditary predisposition to CVID. Neal, my grandfather, died at seventy-six years of age, and I know his cause of death, because I remind myself of it every time I travel by plane. He and my stepgrandmother, Elaine, were traveling to Egypt on vacation when their airliner, EgyptAir Flight 990, was flown into the Atlantic Ocean sixty miles south of Nantucket. After the captain had excused himself to use the head, the relief first officer, Gameel Al-Batouti, uttered, "Tawkalt ala Allah" (I rely on God), and flew the airliner into the Atlantic, killing my grandfather, stepgrandmother, and everybody else on board. It is a reminder: ideas really do matter, and personal

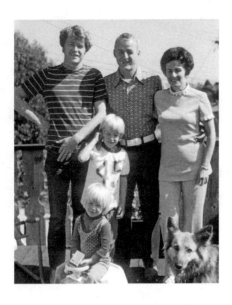

My father, Nelson (*top left*), with my grandfather Neal and his second wife, Elaine, with me and Aaron in Mill Valley, California

convictions do, too—they can justify flying an airliner full of people into the Atlantic, for example.

In the end, my analysis of the Walker and Nelson families indicates that they are not responsible for my CVID. I know far less about the Nelsons because they disappeared into Sweden and have proven hard to track. But the Walkers have been in the United States since the first colonies settled at Plymouth. With the exception of Jeremiah, most Walkers appear to have lived to their historical life expectancy, many much longer. The Walkers have good genes. There were some early deaths in the Nelson family of my paternal grandmother, but no patterns that would suggest something hereditary. But I have never really suspected that my hereditary predisposition for CVID came from my father's side of the family. Even though contemporary descriptions of acquired CVID portray it as largely a spontaneous disease, with autosomal (non-sex chromosomal) origins, Janeway remained convinced that the disease migrated through the maternal side of the family.

CHAPTER 6

Histories

W HEN THE ENVELOPE ARRIVED FROM BENEFIS
Hospitals in Great Falls, I took it from the mailbox and
brought to my office, where it sat unopened for several days. I
had not forgotten about it. I was still curious about what was
inside. But I was also uneasy about opening it. As a Benefis
record-keeper had told me in advance, the envelope contained
the final medical records of my maternal grandfather, LeRoy
Belote, and cursory information about the cause of death of his
twenty-two-year-old sister, Irene. Other members of the Belote
family had also died relatively young in Great Falls, but their
records were lost. I knew that reading through these records
would prove the most wrenching part of this entire project,
even more difficult than reading Charles Janeway's clinical
descriptions of dying children.

Though these medical records served as documentary
sources for my family history of illness, they had once been,

when doctors first communicated the results to my grandfather in January 1976, his death sentence. Not unlike Paul Kalanithi's diagnosis of terminal lung cancer told in *When Breath Becomes Air*, they implied that my grandfather would die before his fifty-sixth birthday; he would die before his dream of living on a farm had been fully realized. I know well the feeling of sitting in a doctor's office, staring at a Pfizer calendar, waiting for blood workup results or radiological interpretations of chest x-rays. I remember well the ensuing discussion about my medical condition, and the basics of my prognosis. "You seem to be doing well, Brett," the doctors always begin. "But if you start to have . . ." is where they generally end. My grandfather often denied that he was ill, according to my mother. He viewed himself as a Montana mountain man, tough and impregnable. But his health challenges caught up with him and swiftly claimed his life. Inside the Benefis envelope were some of the trickiest sources I had ever handled, and I was in no rush to dive into them.

These medical records represented a new kind of source for me. They are sensitive, but not "top secret" like certain state documents; they are not the kind of documentation obtained through a Freedom of Information Act request, for example. They are highly empirical and also interpretative; but a medical specialist, such as a radiologist, interprets them, and they are used to determine what is happening out of sight, inside the human body. They explain discomfort or symptoms; presumably, there was a reason why my grandfather went to the doctor in the first place—bodily pain, for example. But such sources also require negotiating with family, because I am not the only one who shares blood with my grandfather; he was my grandmother's husband, too. They are also different in regard to what they tell the historian. To this point, I have told family stories that largely occurred outside the bodies of my forebearers, events that were externally, rather than internally, experienced by them. Of course, these external experiences, the ones we are "thrown" into, are the experiences that make up the over-whelming bulk of conventional histories: most histories narrate what we do in the outside world, visible for all to see.

Historians value these visible stories of will, agency, and self-determination. In the case of my family history of illness, these stories that occurred externally to the body included William Walker's settlement of Cape Cod, the Walker boys serving as Plymouth Colony freemen, Neal Victor Walker's work for an anti-Catholic newspaper in Missouri, and Neal and Elaine Walker's deaths at the hands of a crazed EgyptAir pilot. I documented these stories and others by mining vital records, newspaper columns, treasury records, draft cards, and death certificates while trying to find evidence of the morbidity and mortality of my relatives. I traced their movement from Eastham to Casper as they sought out business and labor opportunities in the West. I then contextualized some of this vital data and other information in known epidemiological patterns, such as within the 1815 "year without a summer," an event that led to wide-spread typhus outbreaks and food shortages in Ireland and New England. Because some Walkers died in clusters in early 1816, I assumed that epidemic disease had killed them, not complications from CVID, but I will never be certain. Regardless, the Walkers survived these and other challenges and continued to reproduce, hurtling inexorably toward my conception and birth in Bozeman, my CVID diagnosis in Minneapolis, and my desire to write this book.

Such instances of disease are not the patterns of a hereditary susceptibility to CVID, however. Rather, they evince epidemiologic or sporadic disease acquisition. It did not require a compromised immune system to die from typhus during the "year without a summer," as New England mortality figures bear out. It is part of my family history of illness in a general sense, but not the sort of information that my physicians had originally sought. They wanted to know about CVID-like immunological patterns in my family; they sought the rough-cut fractal consistencies created by persistent mortality among blood descendants, preferably ones within three generations. In this regard, such archival evidence brings us only so far, and we now need to transition from standard documentary archives to a blood archive, the documentation of what occurred inside my grandfather's body. The blood archive documents what he felt, what was happening inside his body, and what the expert eyes of doctors saw and communicated to him.

Searching archives for empirical sources is instrumental to writing good history. While researching this book, I spent countless hours in six of Harvard's numerous libraries, including the Countway Library of Medicine, where I researched Janeway's scientific contributions, and the Houghton Library, where rare books are housed. Each one of these libraries proved a valuable source of primary and secondary information about my family history of illness, and each proved instrumental in crafting my medical narrative. I also researched at the Boston Children's Hospital Archives, where I thumbed through another cache of Janeway's personal papers. At the Massachusetts Historical Society archives, I uncovered fragments about the early Walkers of New England. The Montana Historical Society archives proved valuable for information about my Montana family, particularly twentieth-century life as a miner around the Sand Coulee coal mine near Tracy. But none of these archives gave me the cold sweats that the blood archive gave me. The blood archive had the potential to tell me what cellular events had occurred in my family's blood. There was something inescapable about the lessons of the blood archive. I had learned from the documentary archive that my grandfather was a contractor, for example; but I could always escape his vocational legacy by becoming something else. I was free to determine my life's career path in this way, to be willful. Today, I am a teacher, not a builder. But I felt like if I learned that my grandfather had a hereditary susceptibility to blood disease, then I might be unable to challenge this destiny, unable to escape it, and unable to assert my free will over my life. The blood archive promised to subsume me, to trump my destiny, to overpower my own story and wrestle control of my history from me. It threatened to take over my narrative, and that prospect frustrated me. I want to be in charge of my story, much like we all do.

I knew my Montana family would be an important part of my family history of illness. I suspected this because of the intangible connection I felt to my grandfather. It was memories of him, not other relatives, that had first come to me in my hospital bed in Minnesota: he constituted the bulk of my neuronal archives of family, particularly the ones surrounding illness and death. That there might be similarities to my own health challenges, ones that had been forgotten in the forty years since his death, worried me. What if what I had requested from Benefis Hospitals became a kind of crystal ball that revealed my own medical future? This is the power of family history: it has the ability to contextualize the present so fully that it provides a window onto the future.

I had contacted a medical-record keeper at Benefis Hospitals. "Five years ago, I was diagnosed with a blood disorder that my doctors believe is hereditary," I explained in my email, "and I have been trying to determine whether others in my family have had a similar condition." I was told that I could access such records because I was a blood relative, but that I needed to have the closest living relative of my grandfather and his sisters sign a release form. It turned out that this person was my ninety-five-year-old grandmother, the matriarch of my Montana family, Frances Dwyer, the proud daughter of Slovenian immigrants. In order to get access to the blood archive, I had to first explain to her my need to understand my family history of illness. "I don't blame you for wanting to know, Brett," she said, surprising me a little. "I can see why you'd want to know what happened to Dad." To this point my family history of illness had relied on written archival documents that pieced together much of my story; yet another important evidentiary piece, outside the documentary and blood archives, would be the oral interviews with my grandmother that I would record.

Over the course of several years, I had sat down with her to talk about my Montana family. In recent years, her exquisite memory had started to fade, the neuronal trees slowly falling to the forest floor of her being and decomposing with age, and I thought it important to preserve her stories while she could still access them. Oral history is an important part of the toolbox of social historians because it grants access to information that otherwise would never be relayed. People like my grandmother do not often write down their life experiences, so such stories are frequently lost. With a digital recorder in hand, I interviewed this near centenarian on many occasions. She is a woman of humble tastes but surprisingly complex memories of her life in Montana.

— . —

Frances Dwyer's father, Joseph Hocevar, emigrated to the United States from the part of the Austro-Hungarian empire that became Yugoslavia around the turn of the century, probably in 1906. After passing through Ellis Island, he traveled to Montana to meet his brother Frank, who owned the Milwaukee Dairy in Great Falls.

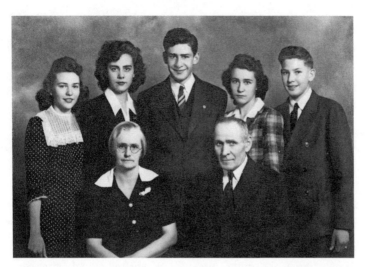

The Hocevar family. My grandmother, Frances, is at far left.

According to Joseph's World War I draft card, he also worked as a meat packer at the Great Falls Meat Company. Frank routinely prodded Joseph to get to know one of the cute Slemberger girls, from another Yugoslavian family, which he did; and in February 1922, wedding bells rang out at St. Ann's Cathedral in Great Falls for Joseph and Frances. They relocated to Tracy, just southeast of Great Falls, where Joseph started work at the Sand Coulee coal mine and where my grandmother was born. As she remembers, Rolly "Bullshit" Brown (she always cackles out loud when she says his nickname) managed the operation for the Great Northern Railroad. Frances was the oldest of five children and was named after her mother and grandmother. "That's how come I love [the name] so much," she giggled.

In Tracy, she fetched pails of drinking water from the Giffin place, cared for the two family dairy cows, and fed the chickens scraps and grains in the yard. "We had a huge garden, but you almost had to with so many kids," she explained. "We had an icebox," she remembered, and the kids relished the ice delivery because they ate the small chips of ice that fell to the floor. "It was just like candy to us," she chuckled. "I delivered milk to the store in lard pails. I can still see them. We also made cream and butter." Then she paused, her impish grin replaced by a more sorrowful countenance. "I can still remember when the chimes would ring when a miner was killed." She never saw the bells, but she remembered their sound as if they had rung yesterday.

Tracy is a small town that once revolved around the Sand Coulee coal mine. Even though Joseph came home from the mines covered in coal dust, my grandmother insisted that "it was a very clean life." During prohibition, Joseph and other Tracy men made moonshine. "They cooked it right there in the kitchen. When the green blinds went down, I knew we was cookin' booze," she laughed. Even the local priest joined in the booze cooking. My grandmother bathed every Saturday evening and always dressed up on Sundays for Catholic service. She recalled every teacher from her Tracy years, including Emilie Wendt, Lillian Nelson, and Bridget Dusak (all names I have confirmed in other histories and documents). But the Sand Coulee coal mine closed down in the 1940s, when the Great Northern Railway transitioned to other fuels; and Joseph took his family back to Great Falls, where he worked in the Anaconda Copper Mining Company works in Black Eagle. Life was not so clean in Great Falls. She remembered that the rental house was an "absolute dump. It was full of bedbugs." But she quickly continued: "I'm sure my folks couldn't afford nothin' else, though, 'cause they never had a dime. . . . Never a dime, Brett." From the Anaconda works in Black Eagle, Joseph brought home chunks of zinc for the kids to melt, pour into molds, and make into toy soldiers. Eventually, with a loan from my grandfather LeRoy, Joseph bought into the Anaconda Commissary, where he worked for the remainder of his life. "By that time he was all crippled up from arthritis," she recalls. "He sure did love that commissary job, though." Joseph knew little in life other than hard labor. He died of lung cancer at seventy-seven years of age.

Most of these Hocevars were healthy people. That Joseph lived seventy-seven years despite having smoked for decades, and after working in the Sand Coulee coal mine and Anaconda smelter in Black Eagle for decades, testifies that he was a man chiseled from granite. Lung cancer eventually got him, but only after years of mine labor. Frances, his wife, did have some health challenges, ones that required her to travel by train in the late 1920s to Rochester to undergo stomach surgery at the Mayo Clinic. After her surgery, Frances lived to be seventy-two years old, easily meeting her twentieth-century historical life expectancy. According to the US Centers for Disease Control and Prevention's *National Vital Statistics Reports*, only about 44 percent of white women lived to see their seventieth birthday in the 1920s. In Joseph's case, he was among the 29 percent of white men to reach seventy-five years of age. So both of my great-grandparents on the Hocevar side exceeded historical life-expectancy norms and are, therefore, not the hereditary source of my CVID.

My grandmother met LeRoy at a dance at the Green Mill Dance Hall in Great Falls. She remembered fondly that Jack Teagarden, an American jazz trombonist, performed with his hard-swinging orchestra. "It was the popular music at the time," she explained, "and it was real music, by the way." (My grandmother has no shortage of strong opinions.) She had attended the dance with another boy, but that did not stop LeRoy from asking her on a date. He had graduated from high school three years earlier, but she had never met him before, even though he had been a jock, playing both baseball and hockey. "I can still remember what dress I had on when he came after me," she remembered. Initially, she coyly responded, "I don't need to go out with you, buddy." But it was not long before the two were cruising Great Falls in his 1939 maroon Buick Coupe. LeRoy worked on construction jobs on the Malmstrom Air Force Base and had a little spare change jingling in his pocket. This was May 1942. My grandmother graduated that June, LeRoy and Frances married in September, and LeRoy left for military training in November. It was an eventful couple of months for the young pair. LeRoy joined the air force and became a pilot, though by the time his training was completed the war was essentially over. LeRoy and Frances spent time in Idaho, Colorado, and Texas while he was in the air force, but they eventually returned to Great Falls after a short stint in Alaska, where Frances broke her back when they dangerously flipped their jeep on the Alaska Highway. Once back in Great Falls, my grandfather started LeRoy O. Belote Construction. Signs in front of his expertly crafted houses read, "When better homes are built, Belote will build them." His father had been a builder, and he would be, too.

But LeRoy really wanted to farm. "He not only wanted to be a farmer," my grandmother lamented, but "he wanted to be on a farm. To live on a farm." He bought land in Cut Bank and near Ulm, but those represented mere stepping-stones for the ultimate goal of buying a large enough farm where he and Frances could live. "He would've had every goddamn animal he could," she recalled. "He had a passion for dogs, a thing for dogs, that you'd not've believed," she explained. "And the thing is, they'd walk and he'd have his hand down and they'd bump his hand to let him know: 'Hey, I'm still here.'" She repeated a sentence, a little embarrassed about her earlier profanity: "He would've had every darn animal he could." But immediately after LeRoy bought the farm, before the ink had even dried on the substantial bank loan, he became seriously ill. "Then, everything went from bad to worse because he found out he had that damn cancer." When he had bought the Cascade farm, he told my grandmother, "I'm not gonna drive another nail, Fran." Of course, farmwork means driving some nails; but it still represented the realization of his lifelong dream, an ancestral blood dream, it turns out; and the realization of that dream corresponded with the death sentence in that Benefis Hospitals envelope in my Cambridge office. His cancer diagnosis caused the transformative gray melancholy that swirled around my family in

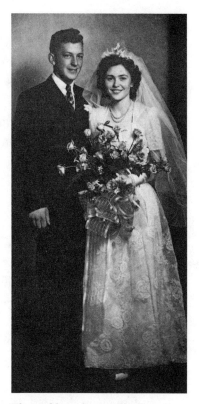

The wedding photograph of my grandparents, LeRoy and Frances Belote, in Great Falls, Montana

the winter of 1975–76. Essentially, it had been created by the contents of that envelope. This is the fall and winter that so defined me. I was a child in a family where the man of the house, an overwhelming presence that had defined manhood for me for years, had just realized a lifelong dream of owning and living on a farm, and then illness had yanked it all away from his strong, calloused hands. Few people could yank anything from those hammer-wielding hands, but disease did. All of this was captured in that envelope.

— · —

It is not surprising that LeRoy wanted to farm. The Belotes were classic American yeoman farmers. They had migrated to the United States from France, where the surname Belot refers simply to an individual from Belleau, Normandy, though my family's name probably hybridized with the English surname Belote in the seventeenth century. They came largely from the Loire Valley region, with its majestic Italian-designed castles, and they lived near Nantes, a city close to Brittany, where many people's ancestors had come from the British Isles. John Belote traveled to Lima, New York, sometime in the early eighteenth century. His son, Isaac Belote, was born in New London, Connecticut, and served in 1759 in the French and Indian War (1755–62) under company commander Captain Nicholas Bishop. The French and Indian War was the North American extension of the Seven Years' War (1755–64), fought between Britain and France. In the nineteenth century, the Belote family began traveling westward, probably following newly laid railroad tracks, looking for opportunities, settling with many other farmers in the northern Ohio River Valley. At the time, life expectancy for men in the United States ranged between sixty-one and eighty years if you saw your twentieth birthday, and the Belote men have a mixed record. Isaac lived to be seventy years old despite combat, but his son, John, died at fifty-six. John's son, John Jr., lived to be seventy-one, but his son, James J., died at forty-seven. Born in New York City, James J. died in Van Buren, Indiana, where the Belote family lived and farmed for several generations before moving to Montana, after a short stint in Michigan.

Like the early Walker family, the members of which sometimes perished in the periodic epidemics that burned through New England settlements, the Belotes faced their own infectious challenges in the nineteenth-century Midwest. In particular, cholera ravaged many of the small towns of Indiana. With my weakened immune system, I would have been toast around cholera, because it is caused by the bacterium *Vibrio cholera* and it attacks the gut. The bacterium colonizes the intestines and sparks symptoms such as diarrhea and vomiting, both leading to dangerous dehydration and electrolyte imbalances. In the Midwest, deadly outbreaks of cholera occurred in 1832, 1849, 1866, and sporadically throughout the 1870s. Because of sanitation challenges, severe cholera outbreaks occurred in large cities such as Saint Louis, Cincinnati, and Detroit, killing in the 1849–51 outbreak as much as 10 percent of the population. But cholera also occurred in many small towns, the kind where members of the Belote family had settled to farm. Small Indiana towns near the Ohio River Valley experienced deadly outbreaks of cholera in the nineteenth century, largely from sewage cesspools leaching into drinking water sources. Often, settlers reacted by simply moving elsewhere. They fled because cholera was part of a spectrum of diseases that physicians associated with damp, unhealthy miasmic air, at least before the advent of the germ theory in medicine. In the minds of settlers, physical environments caused disease, and people sought drier, healthier places in response to epidemics. In 1832, the physician Daniel Drake warned readers of the *Cincinnati Chronicle* that, even though it had "pleased Providence to afflict us with pestilence," Hoosiers do have the "observations of others to guide us" in fighting the deadly disease. Of course, "no one should get drunk," but equally important was that people "should avoid the rain and night air, keep our rooms dry with fires, lodge warm, and dress, as much as possible, in woolens." He then emphasized that "no one, on any account, should neglect the *lax or disordered bowels*," which heralded the onset of cholera and other gastrointestinal illnesses. Nowhere does Drake suggest that people should avoid feces-laced drinking water and its accompanying bacteria, however. This is because Louis Pasteur and Robert Koch were just emerging on the medical scene at this time, and the germ theory did not begin to gain traction until the 1890s.

Often, Ohio River Valley physicians misdiagnosed other internal disorders as cholera, including the mysterious "milk sickness," which settlers later learned was poisoning by the white snakeroot plant. Milk sickness went by many names, including "puking fever," "swamp sickness," and "the slows." It was actually caused by an unsaturated alcohol called tremetol, which the plant harbors in its stems and leaves. It killed a surprising number of farmers in the nineteenth century. Essentially, tremetol resembles turpentine, and when cattle grazed the plant they passed along the poison through milk and milk products. In cattle, the disease was called the "trembles," and symptoms included shaking, stiffness, and collapsing. In people, the symptoms included vomiting and listlessness, as well as ketoacidosis (high concentrations of ketone bodies), hypoglycemia (low blood glucose), lipemia (high lipid blood content), and eventually coma and death. Tremetol causes painful pathological changes within the blood, specifically acidosis (excessive blood acidity), as well as deterioration of the mucosal lining of the stomach, the intestines, liver, kidney, and brain. Drake also weighed in on milk sickness, with about the same level of accuracy as in his observations regarding cholera. In 1838, after John Rowe, an Ohio farmer, killed some of his cattle by experimentally feeding them white snakeroot, he announced his frontier findings in a local newspaper. Drake was quick to pounce and put the Ohio bumpkin in his place. "A professional scrutiny only can be relied on in such cases," he wrote. "The testimony adduced by Mr. Rowe is, therefore, defective and inconclusive." Conclusions about the causes of milk sickness should be left in the hands of professional physicians.

In 1852, the combination of cholera, milk poisoning, and other diseases led the Indiana General Assembly to clear the way for the establishment of boards of health throughout the state. The general assembly also established the Indiana State Medical Society. In his 1878 address, the president of the Indiana State Medical Board, Luther D. Waterman, a prominent Civil War surgeon, emphasized, "We must not cease our labors, as a body, until the citizens of this State have pure air to breathe, pure water to drink, unadulterated food and medicines," and until they "live in buildings that are not sources of infection to themselves or their neighbors." Despite these efforts, however, Indiana settlers often fled the state in the wake of cholera outbreaks in search of healthier environments. Jefferson M. Belote, James J. Belote's son, and his wife, Sara Jennette Gunthorpe, spent their lives in the Midwest, but their son, Lloyd Franklin Belote, pulled up his Midwestern stakes and eventually moved to Montana. He married Lena Odden, from a Norwegian family that had immigrated to Minnesota, and they had several children along the way. Some of their daughters, including Irene, were born in Devil's Lake, North Dakota, as they slowly made their way to Montana's agrarian promised land.

— . —

Lloyd Franklin was born three years after a combined Lakota, Northern Cheyenne, and Arapaho force defeated the Seventh Calvary Regiment of the US Army at Little Bighorn in 1876. But any sense of native euphoria would have been short-lived. The defeat only hardened the US Army's resolve to control the Montana Territory. Immediately after Little Bighorn, Congress increased the maximum size of the army and constructed two

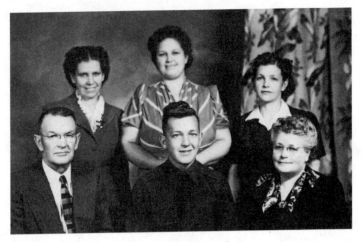

My Belote family. My grandfather LeRoy is at bottom center.

forts to fortify the army's presence in Montana. Fort Keogh, completed in 1877, was on the future Northern Pacific main line, and Fort Custer near Hardin, completed in 1894, was on the future Burlington Route. Lloyd Franklin and Lena would have taken the Great Northern Route, which rumbled past Fort Assiniboine and linked Great Falls to the Midwest in 1887. In such forts, the US Army had stationed thousands of soldiers to protect the "sodbusters" who sought to establish farms in Montana. The two made their way toward the western part of Montana and settled in Dutton, in Teton County, just east of Chouteau. "Chouteau County, they called it," explained my grandmother. "Dad was born in a farmhouse in Chouteau County." Lloyd Franklin and Lena "had what they called a homestead," she told me. It turns out that the key ingredients for bringing the Belote family to Montana were the railroad and the homestead boom of the early twentieth century.

After the Civil War, railroad companies began focusing their attention on westward expansion. Western boosters learned that bringing the railroad to their small towns would sustain their economic growth, and these perennial optimists plied their talents to lure the railway to their doorsteps. In Montana, the mining boom enticed railroad companies, who laid new track well into the twentieth century. Railroads arrived in Montana from three directions. By 1873, the Northern Pacific had reached the Missouri River at Bismarck, North Dakota. The financier of the project, Jay Cooke, had overextended himself, however, and the collapse of his bank caused the Panic of 1873. Railroad construction screeched to a halt. And without the Northern Pacific, as the *Bozeman Times* lamented in 1873, Montana threatened to be a "dull monotonous Territory, cut off from the world and civilization." In 1880, with the Northern Pacific mired in bankruptcy, the Utah and Northern Railroad first reached the Montana Territory line from the south, laying track to Dillon. One year later, the Utah and Northern reached Butte and its potential bonanza of mineral riches. Throughout 1882 and 1883, the Northern Pacific, after substantial reorganization, moved into Montana from both the east and west, hoping to turn Portland, Oregon, into a major hub. The final spike that linked the two was driven in Gold Creek, between Drummond and Deer Lodge. Then, in 1889, the Great Northern Railway Company entered Montana from the north and controlled the coalfields near Tracy, where Joseph Hocevar swung his pick as a coal miner.

By the late 1880s, Montana Territory was crisscrossed with railway lines, which led to an expansion of the mining industry. Although most of the early miners in Montana Territory had focused on gold, miners now turned their attention to silver as well. Montana's first silver discovery occurred in 1864, near Bannack; and with the arrival of investor Marcus Daly in Butte in August 1876, silver mining in Montana Territory underwent a dramatic expansion. In 1880, the territory had produced about 7 percent of the silver in the United States. But once track was laid, Montana became the second-largest producer of silver, with an annual output worth over $20 million. As a result, the demand for other metals also increased, and zinc, lead, gold, and other desirable metals departed Montana in the endless lines of train cars. With the booming economy serving as a powerful tailwind, delegates produced a constitution in 1889 and the territory's voters overwhelmingly approved it. Shortly thereafter, in November 1889, Montana became the forty-first state.

Even more important than Montana's mining boom was its agricultural boom, which was fueled by the Homestead Act (1862). Until 1900, maps labeled the arid region around the Rocky Mountains the "Great American Desert," and most farmers considered the region far too dry for agriculture. But advances in scientific agriculture, particularly dry-farming techniques and mechanical technologies, as well as generous federal land policies — where land was essentially taken from Indians and given to white settlers — led to the homestead boom in Montana. Sodbusters filed some 114,620 homestead claims between 1909 and 1923. One of these individuals was Lloyd Franklin Belote, who settled north of Great Falls near the Golden Triangle, so-called because of its endless sea of ripening wheat fields. Lloyd Franklin was a practitioner of the dry-farming techniques developed by such promoters as Hardy Webster Campbell. Campbell was a South Dakota farmer who maintained that dry farming, or what he called "scientific soil culture," could be just as productive as irrigated farming, and he carefully perfected the Campbell System to preserve moisture content in the soil. Really, the original Homestead Act of 1862 had had little impact on the Montana Territory, because the 160 acres promised to all American citizens proved far too little to be viable in the arid west. In addition, potential homesteaders worried that Native Americans might still force settlers to pay dearly for their land. But immediately after the Battle of the Little Bighorn, the Desert Land Act (1877), which sold 640-acre sections at bargain-basement prices, as well as the Enlarged Homestead Act (1909) and Three-Year Homestead Act (1912), further incentivized farmers to settle in the Great American Desert. When combined with the intensive promotional campaigns that began in earnest in 1908, the boosters proved effective enough to lure Lloyd Franklin and Lena out of the Midwest and into Montana. By 1910, about when Lloyd Franklin claimed his homestead in Dutton, agriculture had surpassed mining as Montana's principal source of revenue.

Natural conditions, too, conspired to lure farmers to Montana. Between 1909 and 1916, Montana's agricultural thirst was quenched—rain seemed to douse dry wheat fields at just the right time. With more than sixteen inches of rain annually, Montana farmers often produced twenty-five bushels an acre. In the "miracle year" of 1915, for example, Montana produced over 42 million bushels of grain. In the Golden Triangle, near where Lloyd Franklin and Lena had settled, farmers occasionally produced thirty-five to fifty bushels per acre annually. After World War I began driving up grain prices, moving to Montana made sense to yeoman farmers, and the state often lived up to its "Treasure State" booster nickname in these years. As my grandmother remembered, Lloyd Franklin even invested in an early mechanical thresher, and other farmers paid for his threshing services. These were the boom years.

Then came drought. The drought started in 1917 along the Hi-Line, in the dry country north of the Missouri River. It did not take long for the drought to spread southward. By 1919, much of Montana was a crunchy, locust-infested nightmare. Forest fires savaged the woodlands, and high winds blew away the topsoil

in Dust Bowl–like conditions. The Campbell System had preserved moisture in the soil, but the deep plowing had loosened
the topsoil layer, which took aloft in the wind, forming swirling
dark clouds. In 1919, the drought reduced the once plentiful
yield of twenty-five bushels an acre to less than two and a half
bushels an acre, and 1920 proved nearly as bad. "They walked
away from it," my grandmother explained. "Nobody wanted to
buy it after what they called the Dust Bowl. They just walked
away." Half of Montana's farmers lost their land in those years.
As this daughter of Slovenian immigrants remembered, it
"kind'a left a bad taste in all those people's mouths."

In Bozeman, I teach in a building named Wilson Hall,
named after M. L. Wilson, a professor of agrarian economics
at the time of Montana's "Dust Bowl" of 1919–20. He is author
of the definitive study of the disaster that cost so many homesteaders so much. "Not every man is a 'natural born' farmer,"
Wilson observed, "but it takes natural born farmers to succeed
at farming." This was particularly true when natural calamities
like severe drought, pests, pockets of poor soil quality, and dam-
aging hail conspire to destroy the dreams of naive sodbusters.
But Wilson concluded that natural calamities did not deserve
all of the blame: many homesteaders, whose backgrounds
ranged from deep-sea diving to wrestling, came to Montana
woefully unprepared for the agrarian task at hand. Over half
of the homesteaders investigated by Wilson came from non-
farming backgrounds, and Montana's punishing conditions
required experienced hands. Lloyd Franklin came to Montana
with considerable farming experience in the Midwest, and he
still went under.

But Lloyd Franklin was a natural farmer, and farming consumed his imagination, even after he took up carpentry in Great
Falls. As my grandmother remembered, "He talked an awful

lot about it. He loved it." I imagine young LeRoy listening to
Lloyd Franklin's family stories of farming. I am sure that while
they pounded nails together, Lloyd Franklin told his son many
stories about farming before the drought of 1919, which had
forced him to abandon his land. He probably told him about
his mechanical thresher, the pride of Dutton. I can see my
grandfather listening intently. I can hear his mind's gears turning. I imagine him, as his hammer strikes another nail, whisper-
ing under his breath: "I'll have a farm of my own someday. I'll
continue that work. I'll show him that it can be done." So after
World War II, as my grandfather built some of the finer homes
in Great Falls, he began buying land. First he bought dry fields
near Cut Bank, and then near Ulm. Then he told Frances, "I'm
not gonna drive another nail, Fran." He bought the big farm in
Cascade, nearly 2,500 acres, and had seven large pivot irrigators
installed. The giant sprinklers would suck water directly from
canals diverted from the Missouri, which snaked near the farm;
they would ensure that his dreams never blew away in a cloud
of dust the way Lloyd Franklin's had. "It was just in their goddamn blood," my grandmother lamented to me.

— · —

I knew none of this in 1997, when I received my PhD from the
University of Oregon and, the next year, began teaching at Yale
University. I had forgotten about the Cascade farm and largely
about my deceased grandfather. I had spent years studying in
Japan and had gained new cosmopolitan perspectives on the
world. My dissertation explored the epidemiological and environmental legacies of the Japanese colonization of the northern
island of Hokkaido, particularly the conquest of the indigenous
Ainu people. Their tragic experiences, it occurred to me, par-
alleled the tragic experiences of Native Americans, such as

those in Montana, and those historical symmetries interested me. I thrived at Yale, particularly enjoying the lively intellectual climate, but colleagues had cautioned me from the outset that Ivy League universities did not often give tenure, and to always be on the lookout for more permanent employment. My first year at Yale, I was alerted to a job in Japanese history that had opened up at Montana State University in Bozeman, and immediately a flood of Montana memories that had been dormant for over a decade began returning. Without warning, the prospect of returning to Montana became a real one, and I found myself revisiting my childhood obsession with the Big Sky State. The next year, my then-wife and I left New Haven for Bozeman and began teaching in the town of my birth. I did not realize it yet, but my return to Montana was about more than just career adjustments. It was also about family and landscape.

By the time I had started teaching at Yale, the vicelike grip of the cultural turn on the discipline of history had started to loosen. In the subfield of environmental history, historians began exploring the idea of building a new "ecological history," one that wed ecological theories of environmental change with a strong commitment to empiricism. The cultural turn had seriously weakened categories such as science, often questioning the basic stability of an empirical fact. With the cultural turn, everything had become subjective, contingent on the race and gender of the observer, and always situated in its unique historical moment or place. Often, the cultural turn had replaced science with historically constructed "sciences," and had replaced facts with subjective "experiences." In contrast, environmental history had tethered its analysis to understanding physical environments through the use of ecological and epidemiological sciences. It focused on how people altered those environments in historical time, as well as how those environments altered people. I was completely seduced in graduate school by the promise of environmental history, as the cultural turn had always felt intellectually unsustainable to me.

In my first book, for example, *The Conquest of Ainu Lands*, I compared the Japanese conquest of Hokkaido to settler colonialism in the U.S. West, in particular the roles of overhunting for trade and of epidemic diseases in undermining Ainu independence. I found the bony skeleton of global comparative structures in this story, one that afforded rich cross-cultural comparisons. Both Native Americans and the indigenous Ainu, even though they lived in completely different contexts, had experienced a ruthlessly similar historical reality, exposing globally consistent rather than locally specific forces in driving colonial settlement. Tuberculosis, for example, killed people no matter their culture, race, or gender. The bacillus that causes tuberculosis lived before its discovery in 1882, existing beyond the subjective experience of Robert Koch, its discoverer, and his social networks and relationships. Such diseases as tuberculosis became less historical categories than independent actors, dangerous bacilli with real influence on history. Donald Worster, a pioneer in the field, insisted that environmental historians sought to integrate into their narratives "autonomous, independent energies that do not derive from the drives and inventions of any culture." That anything could exist outside of "any culture" was intellectually inconceivable in the logic of the cultural turn, as everything was historically and culturally situated, even the tuberculosis bacillus. But after a childhood spent outdoors, either on the Montana farm or in the Cascade Mountains, I was attracted to the physical aspect of Worster's thinking. Growing up, I had always preferred raccoon tails and cat skulls to books, and environmental history afforded me the opportunity to investigate both.

Entrenched opposition to Worster's thinking already existed in the discipline of history, however, and that opposition was situated in earlier debates over what constituted agency. R. G. Collingwood, a British philosopher and historian, had written that only political thinking drove history, because everything else, such as Worster's "autonomous, independent energies," was natural and, therefore, fell outside the scrutiny of the historian's lens. For Collingwood, the actual thought process of the historical subject remained critical, much as it had for Leopold von Ranke, and the historian's task was to "reenact" that thought process through the use of "historical imagination." It was impossible for historians to get inside the tiny head of a bacillus, and not only because they do not really have heads. Collingwood wrote, "The right way of investigating nature is by the methods called scientific," while "the right way of investigating mind is by the methods of history." This separation of natural and historical spheres also characterized both Ranke's and Edward P. Thompson's approaches to the discipline. Collingwood asserted that there is a difference between "timefulness," what he defined as simply change over time, and history proper. History is change over time in relation to "human affairs," because the "events of nature are mere events, not the acts of agents" who drive historical progress through conscious action. In other words, there was a real possibility that environmental historians did not study history at all, because it was difficult to call a bacillus a historical agent.

Similarly, Marc Bloch, a French social historian and cofounder of the Annales School, cautioned that "we must beware of postulating any false geometric parallels between the science of nature and a science of man." Like Collingwood, he separated the medical sciences from history, writing that the "biologist may indeed study respiration, digestion, or the motor functions

separately; for all that, he is not unaware that there is a whole person for which he must account." He continued: "The difficulties
of history are of still another nature. For in the last analysis it
is human consciousness which is the subject-matter of history."
Like Collingwood, Bloch envisioned history as seeing "through"
the human subject in order to retrieve the mechanisms of historical choices. He wrote that the "interrelations, confusions, and
infections of human consciousness are, for history, reality itself."

For his part, Collingwood was concerned with the "inside"
life of the mind, and he peered "through" events in the past
to see their inner meaning, not "at" them, which allowed one
only to describe "bodies and their movements." In this Cartesian framework, historians should not concern themselves with
"respiration, digestion, or the motor functions" of the body,
only the intricacies of cognition and consciousness. By Collingwood's and Bloch's definitions, then, my family history of illness falls short of the threshold of history because it looks at
"outside" natural events and the "inside" mechanisms of the
body—the morbidity and mortality of family members as they
lived and died in "timefulness" chronology—and does not see
"through" their conscious actions. My family history of illness is
largely about "bodies and their movements." By the traditional
definitions of Ranke, Collingwood, Bloch, and even Thompson, a family history of illness is not really possible because it is
not history in the sense that it "reenacts" the past. Why would
anyone want to reenact disease and death anyway? These are
among the most natural of all processes.

But what if the "inside" that historians investigate constituted more than just thought processes inside the mind? What
if the mind was not exclusively in charge of thinking? What if
the "inside" that historians look at included Sherrington's "the
material me"—the workings of the body's viscera and central

nervous system—and the manner in which it drove my behavior, choices, and even conscious actions? What if my body, and its microbial communities, became the historical "inside" and agents of my choices? It is counterintuitive, but my family history of illness, which has stretched from Janeway's research to my family's migration across the country, has entailed as much "big history" as it has microhistory, because I have sought to identify the "ordered patterns that appear at all scales" in our bodies and beyond, such as the points I made about proteins and memory. I have sought patterns throughout this entire narrative, including those of blood proteins and neuronal forests, as well as B-cells, the biological architecture of memory, and historians and their archives.

Historian David Christian has written that "big history" is interested in "ordered entities, from molecules to microbes to human societies to large chains of galaxies," because whether "chemical in the case of molecules" or "biological in the case of microbes," some "principles of change may be universal." Scientists and historians are interested in these ordered patterns because people are "pattern-detecting organisms," whether those patterns include "galaxies and stars, the chemical elements, the solar system, our earth, and all the living organisms that inhabit our earth." It was this search for patterns that drove Benoit Mandelbrot to discover fractal geometry and to search for patterns in the most unlikely places, such as the coastline of the British Isles or in tumultuous financial markets. Reticent to acknowledge that he "invented" anything, including the Mandelbrot set, he explained that such rough patterns exist and wait to be observed. The Mandelbrot set "has always been there, but a particular life orbit made me the right person at the right place at the right time to be the first to inspect this object," he mused. The patterns themselves are not figments of the cultural imagination, they actually exist independent of mind, but culture and history determined the overwhelming context that allowed Mandelbrot to "inspect" them. This is what I think historians do as well—they inspect the past through interrogation of the sources, certainly as much as they invent it with their theoretical imagination.

Inspecting patterns is an important part of our evolutionary tool kit that has allowed us to survive. According to Christian, life, as opposed to lifeless matter, is built from "proteins that dominate the chemistry and the structure of all living organisms" and is more complex than anything else in the universe. "Collectively," he wrote, "living organisms explore their environment in ways that have no parallel in the inanimate world. And what they find is new sources of energy and new ways of organizing themselves so as to survive the hurricane of energy flowing through them." The complexity of life is a natural extension of these energy-seeking patterns, as are the nutrient- and warmth-seeking bacteria that inhabit my body. Of all aspects of our complexity, human language sets us apart from other forms of life most strikingly. Individuals can "deliberately think about the past and imagine the future" and, in doing so, create a "common pool of ecological and technical knowledge" that people pass down through time in the form of history. Big history is all about transporting the reader through vertigo-inducing scales. Christian argued that elaborate patterns exist throughout history—from molecules and cells, from the earliest agricultural communities to the most complex states, and from stars and galaxies. It is up to historians to uncover and inspect them.

Inspecting such rough patterns has become a hallmark of environmental history, including what is called evolutionary history and neurological deep history. Edmund Russell, a proponent of evolutionary history, has his eyes on big patterns, particularly those patterns that demonstrate how human history intersects with biological evolution. He has sought to dispel the misconception that evolution is something that happens "out there," separate from people in both time and space. Because humans are deeply embedded in the earth's natural systems, our decisions drive evolution in the natural world. Not only do my diet and the strength of my immune system shape my microbial communities but so, too, do other historical forces, such as the pervasive use of antibacterial soaps. Of course, using antibacterial soaps during the cold and flu seasons seems wise, but antibacterial soap often contains an ingredient called triclosan. Makers of these soaps advertise that they kill 99 percent of the bacteria they encounter. But as Russell speculates, with millions of bacteria living on and in our bodies, the cultural practice of handwashing is driving the natural evolution of microbial communities. Bacteria evolve defensive traits that protect them against triclosan, and such traits also make them resistant to antibiotics. It turns out that triclosan-resistant bacteria survive the formidable onslaught of our most powerful antibiotics, including the ones that saved me in the Minneapolis hospital. There is triclosan in our bodies, as many manufacturers put it in toothpaste, mouthwash, deodorants, toys, and plastic kitchenware. "Our bodies are environments for the bacteria that live in and on them, and the products we use affect that environment," observed Russell. He added that, the "wealthier you are, the more likely you are selecting for triclosan-resistant bacteria." Wealthier people often buy more expensive personal care products, more of which contain triclosan.

These bacteria become culturally constructed, but not in the manner that the cultural turn might have viewed them. These bacteria are culturally constructed because they have evolved as a result of people's consumer choices, which is affecting "the material me" in a number of ways. But the structure of

Russell's evolutionary history is a global one: antibiotic-resistant bugs are killing people in droves in the United States, China, and Vietnam, to name just the cases he discusses. These bugs are not subjective figments of the cultural imagination. Rather, they are Worster's "autonomous, independent energies," independent living entities that operate both within and without our cultures, and within and without our bodies as well. They are cultural constructs in an evolutionary way, not purely as figments of the imagination.

Daniel Lord Smail, a Harvard historian, has also sought to inspect some of the rough patterns of historical experience, but in the context of the deepest recesses of the evolutionary history of the brain. Collingwood had insisted that historians see "through" the conscious actions of their subjects, and what better way than to focus on the organ most responsible for that consciousness. Not unlike big historian David Christian, deep historian Smail is principally concerned with scales of time, particularly the "point of rupture, the moment in time, in or around the fourth millennium B.C.," when cultural humans replaced biological ones. With the ascendance of culture, humans began creating civilizations; and with those early states came written documents; and in this context history began. Even though sporting a brain about the same size as mine, that earlier biological human, with its protruding forehead and hairy shoulders, has been left to other academic disciplines. Smail seeks to bring that earlier biological human and its brain into contemporary history, by linking "features of culture" with "human physiology." By doing so, he identifies the importance of "human sameness as well as cultural difference." Smail's emphasis on "sameness" is important, because these represent the same rough patterns that lead to the erection of new structures and comparative frameworks in the discipline of history. For example, as I have argued elsewhere, if medieval feudalism in western Europe looks similar to that in Japan, as it most assuredly does, with knights in one and samurai in the other, then either this is weirdly coincidental, because there was no sustained contact between Europe and Japan, or there is a neurohistorical reason for this example of parallel development. With neurohistory, Smail has sought to liberate the study of history from the time lines of the national and the sacred, and the intellectual laziness of the coincidental, instead placing people in a more comparative biological time line.

Smail rejects Collingwood and others and aligns more with Heidegger, Mandelbrot, Worster, and Russell, stating, "I do not hold with the idea that a consciousness of history is a prerequisite for historicity, preferring to join with others in believing that history is something that *happens* to peoples, things, and organisms, and is not *made* by them." Smail's observations are important for me because they rescue my family history of illness from the dustbin of Ranke's historical wannabes. Smail pointed out that there is much at stake with policing the "point of rupture" between biological and cultural human, because the emergence of writing remains one of the hallmarks of what the French historian François Guizot referred to as the "superiority of man over all other creatures." To bring the biological human into today's world risks wrenching the cultural human back into the ranks of the animal kingdom. Smail insisted that history's privileging of the written word over other artifacts of memory needlessly limits the historian. More broadly, memory has always served as an "archival and historical medium in Postlithic societies," and memory more broadly, rather than just written documentation, should be the principal interest. Memory bears directly on human cultural evolution, which is, much like our modulating immune systems, a product of epigenetics. By transmitting learned information to new generations through teaching history, people have accelerated the rate of change in our species.

Smail drags history kicking and screaming back to the African savanna, where the bulk of the human brain evolved, which allowed "individuals to negotiate the escalating complexities posed by human social living"—in other words, the central nervous system is universal to the human species. As Smail wrote, "The existence of brain structures and body chemicals means that predispositions and behavioral patterns have a universal biological substrate that simply cannot be ignored. This is the principle that lies behind the neurohistorical approach." Among other predispositions, this biological approach "demands that we acknowledge a genetic and behavioral legacy from the past," an assumption that drives the basic idea of a family history of illness. The "biological substrate" that Smail referred to is one more example of the new structures being inspected by recent historians.

Timothy LeCain, a colleague of mine at Montana State University and a self-proclaimed "neo-materialist" historian, has taken the historical examination of the role of the physical and biological world in driving human affairs to new heights in *The Matter of History*. By exploring the molecular composition of copper, the ecologies of silkworms and cattle, the microorganisms in our stomachs, and other material things that shape our world, LeCain takes aim at the entire notion of human-centered history, particularly that framed by the geologic Anthropocene epoch. "If this age has anything to teach us," he wrote of the Anthropocene, "it may well be that humans are not in control, that we do not create our world in any conscious sense but are swept along by powerful material things that we only dully comprehend. Humans may appear to be the dominant species of the moment, yet it is because the planet we pretend to dominate has made us so."

For LeCain, as much as we live in an age dominated by human cognition and consciousness, class and economy, and subjective identity-forming experiences such as gender and race, we also live in an "age of coal and steel, of oil, an age of cows and silkworms, cotton and copper, and age of corn and rice: we live in an age of sulfur, of arsenic and asbestos, an age of diethylstilbestrol and bis-phenols." Moreover, he noted, we live in an age of "hard concretes and soft plastics and sharp, shiny aluminum, and an age of bright electric lights that erase the infinite stars from our eyes. This supposed Age of Humans is all of these *things* and many more, but never just human, because these are the very things that have made us human." If the discipline of history began in the nineteenth century with Ranke's pursuit of "pure perception" through the study of primary sources, and then later entailed Collingwood's twentieth-century attempt to "reenact" past thought processes through the use of "historical imagination," then it has arrived in the twenty-first century with LeCain's assertion that "much of what makes us so deeply and uniquely human comes not from within us but from the organisms and things around us."

The important point is that history is *happening* everywhere all the time, not necessarily *created* by the willful hands of a small cohort of lucky souls. From the rubble of the weakened structures of social history, environmental historians have created a new material structure, one, at least as I've portrayed it in this book, cobbled together with the physical world that swirls around us, as well as with the biological substrate of our shared brains and bodies. In this way, my family history of illness is as much about typhus and cholera contagions, train engines and railroad tracks, horses and military forts, disappearing Indian bodies and multiplying white ones, anti-Catholic newspapers and mechanical threshers, industrial environments saturated in chemicals and heavy metals, genotypes and phenotypes, and blood disorders and collapsing immune systems as it is about what any members of my family thought as they migrated, some across the United States, others across the world, to Montana. Importantly, the story of one of those bodies was in that Benefis Hospitals envelope, and it was time to open it.

— · —

I had asked Benefis Hospitals for the medical records of my grandfather LeRoy, as well as of his three sisters, out of four, who had died relatively young: Irene, Ethel Geneviere, and Hazel. My grandmother had explained that nearly all of LeRoy's sisters had died young of cancer. The Benefis Hospitals records regarding Irene were confined to some barely legible notes scribbled into a larger record book, which included notes on other patients. The brief notation listed her address (322 Fourth Street North, where her family lived, according to the 1930 and 1940 US Census), her date of birth (September 7, 1911), her occupation (waitress), her doctor (Dr. Richardson), and her examination room (Room 441). She "expired" on July 23, 1933. According to her records, Dr. Richardson had diagnosed Irene with three dangerous blood conditions that were probably interrelated. But other than that, the records are bare-boned. He first listed agranulocytosis (also known as agranulosis or granulopenia), which is an acute form of leukopenia (lowered white blood cell counts) that leaves patients at risk of infections, depending on the degree to which the white blood cells counts are diminished. Often, agranulocytosis means low neutrophil counts, the body's most numerous kind of white blood cells (or granulocytes), but the disease can also be characterized by inadequate eosinophil and basophil numbers. Not unlike my CVID, agranulocytosis heightens the patient's risk of bacterial and fungal infections, but the kinds of infections differ. Although pneumonia and septicemia (blood infection) are symptoms shared by CVID and agranulocytosis, cellulitis (infections on the skin or just below the surface of the skin), liver abscesses, and furunculosis (deep infection of a hair follicle leading to an abscess) are, to my knowledge, not shared symptoms. In his research, for example, Janeway had determined that CVID also led to bacterial infections, including pneumonia and septicemia, but not the skin infections caused by agranulocytosis.

As far as the Benefis Hospital record-keeper could make out, Dr. Richardson also diagnosed Irene with "acute lymphangitis," which is often caused by an acute streptococcal infection of the skin and might have been related to the agranulocytosis. Finally, Dr. Richardson diagnosed her with leukemia, a disorder that begins when the bone marrow produces abnormal white blood cells, known as blasts or leukemia cells. There are different kinds of leukemia, but Dr. Richardson offered no details. Importantly, medical researchers believe that both hereditary and environmental factors are involved with the onset of leukemia, and it is impossible to tell what caused Irene's cancer specifically. But something awful had happened to her at a very young age, and the pretty waitress from Great Falls, before she could really get a start on life, died of blood cancer at twenty-two. Needless to say, this revelation, that she had an immune problem and had developed leukemia, scared me. But Irene's was not the same disease. With CVID, I do not necessarily have a diminished number of white blood cells; mine just stopped producing antibodies in response to bacterial infection. I share with Irene an immunological disorder, but one of a different variety. The relationship is intriguing, but medically inconclusive.

LeRoy's medical story was different, however. I was sent nearly twenty pages on my grandfather. On January 4, 1976, LeRoy was admitted to the hospital because of fainting spells, a mediastinal mass in his chest, and known diabetes mellitus, which had first been diagnosed in 1967. While he was in the hospital in January, his diabetes was "under control," wrote his physician Dr. F. J. Allaire, a University of Michigan–educated internal specialist. But after careful examination, doctors discovered lacunar infarcts (signs of a stroke that occurs from occlusion of one of the brain's main arteries), which is sometimes associated with diabetes. While hospitalized in January, he underwent a battery of invasive tests, including an aortic arch study, a carotid and vertebral angiography, a cytology, a right supraclavicular lymph node excision, a transfemoral route angiography, sinus x-rays, chest x-rays, urinalysis, and a series of comprehensive blood tests. It must have been awful. The final diagnosis was deadly serious, though: diabetes mellitus, squamous cell carcinoma, metastasis to mediastinum, and lacunar infarcts. My interpretation of his first admission record from Montana Deaconess Hospital is that he had diabetes and cancer of the epithelial wall of his lungs, which had metastasized to the lymph nodes in his chest cavity. He also had suffered through some minor strokes, most likely as a result of his diabetes.

The next admission record is dated a little over a month before his death, on September 16, 1976. "The patient was admitted for management of weakness," Dr. Allaire begins. "It was found that the diabetes mellitus was somewhat out of control also." He was diagnosed with "mild ketosis without acidosis," which is elevated ketones in the body caused by abnormal fat metabolism, also associated with diabetes. The doctors gave him forty-five units of lente insulin (an intermediate-acting insulin) daily, plus regular insulin, procaine penicillin (a slow-acting antibiotic), and Dimetane expectorant (to relieve coughing). Doctors also treated him with Bronkosol and a nebulizer. His sputum culture showed "normal throat flora," suggesting that his immune system continued to function even while under assault by lung cancer and irradiation therapy. Another physician, Dr. Lenz, gave my grandfather penicillin V potassium, five hundred milligrams; Dulcolax suppositories; and more insulin. The final diagnosis remained deadly serious: diabetic ketoacidosis, right middle-lobe pneumonia, left lower-lobe pneumonia, carcinoma of the lung.

During my grandfather's September hospitalization, Dr. Allaire drafted a brief history of his health challenges. He started by explaining, "This patient has been going downhill for the last month with progressive anorexia and [an] inability or unwillingness to drink enough fluids." It seems that the "patient," my grandfather, was for some reason "unwilling" to drink enough fluids, and that he had progressively become anorexic. In one conversation with my grandmother, I asked how LeRoy had handled his diabetes diagnosis. She explained, "Oh, it was a big adjustment for the both of us, not just him. We tried to find out if it was in the family, but didn't have much luck." Over time, they discovered that "you can still live and have a halfway decent life, . . . but you had'a take care of yourself." She noted that "he had to boil all his old needles . . . everything. . . . It was a mess. He had his own little system. His own little pan to boil things in." Regarding his cancer diagnosis, I asked if doctors had understood his lung cancer to be caused by smoking cigarettes. He had probably smoked for thirty years. "Yeah, very definitely that," she answered. "If he wouldn't've smoked, he wouldn't've have had cancer." Even after his cancer diagnosis in January 1976, he continued to go for walks at night to smoke cigarettes. "He thought he was foolin' everybody, but he wasn't," she said of his nightly walks. When I asked her if the cancer was an aggressive one, she answered, "I'm sure it was. . . . He was toast . . . and he was still smokin'." When I asked if he had been unwilling to drink fluids in the hospital, she answered, "That wouldn't surprise me," as if he were sitting right next to her.

In 1967, Dr. Allaire continued, physicians had first diagnosed LeRoy with brittle-type diabetes, a particularly hard-to-control form of type 1 diabetes. He had had several bouts of recurring ketoacidosis as a result, including in 1970, 1971, and late 1975. My grandfather had started complaining of the lacunar infarcts in early 1976, with neurological symptoms including general "weakness" and partial paresthesia of the right leg. His first cancer diagnosis had been in January. Then, doctors had determined it to be inoperable based on a lymph node "practically completely replaced by well-differentiated squamous cell carcinoma." He did receive cobalt irradiation, but with little result. He continued to see Dr. Taylor, who had conducted the supraclavicular lymph node excision, and other doctors over the summer, but his condition only worsened. Dr. Allaire concluded his report by explaining, "He is not drinking well, not eating well and will be admitted to the hospital." After this admittance, he never left.

The "very thin white male," as he was described in one report, only got worse. He had progressive dyspnea (cardiovascular disease), and there was an "alveolar spread of his carcinoma," which was "corroborated by positive sputum cytology." Experts checked his skull, his lumbar spine, and his pelvis and conducted a "total body bone scan." His liver and spleen worked, and his sigmoidoscopy (a procedure that enables a view inside the sigmoid colon and rectum) showed nothing irregular. His echocardiogram was normal. He had a brain scan and a cerebral flow study, and the results were normal. But his lung cancer continued to worsen. On October 15, a radiologist, Dr. H. N. Mazjurkiewicz, noted his impressions of the x-rays: "The most likely diagnosis would be lymphatic spread of the patient's known carcinoma with superimposed areas of either pulmonary edema or infiltrate migrating throughout different portions of the lung fields." By mid-October, my grandfather's cancer was spreading out of control. On October 22, another radiologist, Dr. Fred M. Long, wrote, "There has been no significant change in the diffuse infiltrating disease since our examination of 10-15-76. There may be a very slight pleural effusion on the right." Then, mercifully, on October 30, LeRoy "quietly expired," as noted by Dr. Allaire. His final diagnosis: "Squamous cell carcinoma of lung with metastasis to mediastinum and left clavicular lymph nodes, Hypercalcemia. Diabetes mellitus."

"We didn't even know that he was sick until the very end," my mother told me. "They never said anything." But this certainly explained the summer of 1976, when we had disassembled the Quonset hut in Great Falls. It was then that he had said, "I know, I'm not supposed to be smoking." What must have been going through his mind while he looked at his little white-headed grandson staring obliviously at his thin silhouette? "It'll be our secret, Brett," he had told me. And, it had been our secret, but only until I became ill myself.

I started my family history of illness in an attempt to bring some context, an explanatory framework, to my own health challenges and, as a result, came to better understand LeRoy's but not necessarily mine. I feel like I finally know him now. He is no longer a phantasm of my childhood Montana dreams, but a real, fleshy person, with a body and blood, and that blood flows through my veins, too. His blood, his history, his dreams run through my body, my mind, and my own story. And while

I still cannot definitively link his illnesses to my own—he appears to have contracted lung cancer by smoking—his legacy continues to drive me in ways that I am only now starting to appreciate. In researching this book, I wanted answers to better understand myself; but maybe I need to heed his advice and sit and wait—soon, "they will come," unlike the elk that never did. My grandfather's medical story has made me appreciate the place of family history in understanding illness, but also its limitations.

Even if it does not fully explain my health challenges, I understand now the nearness of his disease. At a basic level, I have disease in my family, but I am not sure I have a family history of illness. In my family, there are incidences of cancer, diabetes, and other serious diseases, but my grandfather's children, including my mother, are healthy as horses. I am left to ponder, then, which is more important: my individual history, the one that made me the environmentally influenced phenotype that I am; or my family's history and the genes I share with my near and distant ancestors? If I am Brett the Phenotype, then my individual agency in life—the places I worked, the environments where I lived, the places I traveled, the choices I made—becomes important in understanding my diagnosis with CVID. This realization, that the individual really does matter, led me to change some of my basic assumptions about how history works. As much as history simply *happens*, perhaps we do *create* it as well, and our bodies are part of that creation process.

Legacies

I N RECENT YEARS, THE CENTERS FOR DISEASE CONTROL and Prevention (CDC) have encouraged people to document their families' health histories with a series of online medical history tools. One such tool is "My Family Health Portrait," which allows an individual to create a family history of illness that extends three generations deep. "Talking with your health provider about your family health history can help you stay healthy!" the text accompanying the online tool states. "Family health history can help your child's doctor make a diagnosis if your child shows signs of a disorder," by demonstrating your child's hereditary susceptibility toward a particular health challenge. "Many genetic disorders first become obvious in childhood," the CDC website explains, "and knowing about a family health history of a genetic condition can help find and treat the condition early."

But the CDC website is quick to caution that "having a family health history of a disease does not mean that your child will get that disease." In other words, a family history of illness best tracks potential problems, mainly congenital ones that manifest symptoms early in life. It is not an absolute determination of anything, however. It is a critical part of any medical decision, not the sole consideration. The portrait generated by the "My Family Health Portrait" tool, the one parents are encouraged to provide to their doctors, is a one-page snapshot populated by immediate family members and their medical conditions. According to "My Family Health Portrait," mine is a healthy family, other than my grandfather on my mother's side. The CDC's portrait tool proved frustratingly inconclusive to me, though it might be helpful in making basic medical decisions for some. To begin with, I do not see history as a portrait of anything. Rather, history is more a braided line than a horizontal plane. It is a braid of happenings and creations that form a narrative, which is laid out in logical, causative order, one that gives meaning to people and events. If one page of that history is removed from its context, say, in the way that a portrait is removed from its context, it says virtually nothing; the happenings and creations all have to be examined together, contextualized by what came before and what came after, to make any sense. In the case of a braided line on a sailboat, once the strands have been fouled, cut, or frayed, the line is essentially worthless; this is also true of cohesive narratives.

The information collected by the tool "My Family Health Portrait" is very different from what I sent my physician, Professor Gregory Vercellotti, in the Division of Hematology, Oncology, and Transplantation at the University of Minnesota. Dr. Vercellotti is a former senior associate dean for education, and he has wide-ranging academic interests. About three months before I finished this book, I sent him a draft of it, a less polished version of the one that you have nearly finished. "I finally have

an answer to your question about my family history of illness," I
wrote him, half joking, but half not, in the accompanying email.
"I actually do not think that I have a family history of illness, at
least not one that would be useful to you in understanding my
CVID diagnosis. But I am interested in hearing what you think."
I was hoping that my book would have clinical value, and that it
would help explain why I was diagnosed with CVID when other
members of my family were not; but now, as I conclude the
project, I am not sure that it does explain my diagnosis. Was the
explanation of my CVID diagnosis in my family history of illness, or did I acquire the disease sporadically—that is, randomly
or accidentally—because of environmental circumstances, in a
manner that I might never fully understand?

As I mentioned, I have disease in my family but am not sure
that this necessarily translates into a family history of illness.
Both sides of my family had navigated the illness-infested waters
of life in colonial America, suffering through the ebbing and
flooding of local and global epidemiological tidewaters. I cannot
be certain, but it is possible that Jeremiah Walker, for example,
who died at thirty-eight years of age, succumbed to an epidemic
that swept through New England. He died in 1740 in Harwich,
possibly as a result of one of the multiple smallpox outbreaks
that hit Massachusetts in the mid-eighteenth century, or a measles outbreak that flared between 1739 and 1741. They are both
killers. As in the case of many such dangerous epidemics, Jeremiah would not have needed a compromised immune system
to succumb to either smallpox or measles, though CVID would
certainly have aided the disease. The extant documents provide
no concrete answers regarding the status of Jeremiah's antibodies; but they do contextualize the epidemiological and medical world he lived within, which is equally helpful. Viewed this
way, the smallpox virus may have been the agent of Jeremiah's

premature death, but the cause was more likely a web of historical factors that brought the agent of death to his body.

Jeremiah's son, Benjamin, lived to see his ninetieth year but then died in 1816, the same year as his son, Marshall, and his daughter-in-law, Hannah. Marshall and Hannah Walker died in their midfifties within a week of one another, strongly suggesting that their deaths related to the eruption of Mount Tambora and the global cooling during the "year without a summer." Global cooling devastated crops and weakened bodily immune systems worldwide, which contributed to epidemiological irruptions. With malnourished bodies spending more time indoors to keep warm, typhus was able to spread among these huddled people, which may have included my kin. Clearly, this kind of textured historical detail would not have fit into the CDC's "My Family Health Portrait," but it remains an important component of my family history of illness, nonetheless. Admittedly, I am speculating here, but the explanation is as plausible as anything else. Without antibiotics or even the germ theory of medicine that spawned antibiotic therapies, families such the early American branch of mine navigated a world haunted by unseen bacteria and viruses. Microbes might as well have been ghosts, because people did not even have the conceptual tools to imagine them or the technological abilities to view them—diseases were still caused by miasmic air. Nonetheless, it was not mountain lions and bears that hunted my colonial American relatives but microbial predators, even if they were not yet known. Similarly, members of the Nelson family, my paternal grandmother's family, died young in Sweden, but my grandmother herself was a sturdy old bird. She had some health problems later in life, including strokes, but they most likely resulted from lifestyle choices, such as smoking cigarettes for many decades. But her experiences, too, which may or may not have any bearing on my medical condition, remain part of my family history of illness. Interestingly, in my family's story there is as much resilience as susceptibility.

Judging from my maternal grandmother's health, the Hocevar family appears to have been as tough as nails. These gritty Slovenian immigrants knew nothing but hard labor but still walked through life with a certain degree of strength and grace. They provided the bedrock for my Montana family as I was growing up. As for the Belote family, there is James J. Belote, whose death in 1865 at forty-seven years of age remains a mystery, but could possibly have been related to one of the periodic cholera epidemics that swept through the northern Ohio River Valley. Other than James and my grandfather, LeRoy, the Belote family mainly met or exceeded their historical life expectancies. My grandfather probably smoked for over thirty years before he died, and my grandmother insists that doctors linked his lung cancer to smoking. The "merchants of doubt" might tell you otherwise, but cigarettes probably killed him. Certainly, his diabetes could have been hereditary, but my grandmother claims that, after his diagnosis, the two briefly researched his family history (at the request of his doctors) to see if anybody had the disease, and could find no evidence of it. It is possible that James J. Belote died of diabetes, but I have no method to determine whether or not he did.

My mother insists that she always believed her father's diabetes was related to his wildly fluctuating eating habits, including his breakneck dieting when he believed he was getting overweight. She often dieted with him. She remembers that it was after he dieted and lost a great deal of weight that his diabetes first manifested. In other words, perhaps the predisposition was there, and maybe James J. Belote did die of diabetes, but lifestyle choices may have triggered the disease. It turns out that heredity is common with type 1 diabetes. Of course, Irene and the other

Belote daughters died young of cancer, and it is entirely possible that, given the right lifestyle or environmental circumstances, members of the Belote family do develop cancer. But as of this writing, my uncle Lee, my aunt Leslie, and my mother are all quite healthy. That a predisposition for cancer runs in the Belote family does not necessarily translate into getting cancer. Again, Belote family members all share genetic similarities, but my grandfather clearly became a different phenotype—that is, an individual resulting from the interaction of genotypes and the environment owing to life experiences and choices.

The CDC acknowledges that lifestyle choices intersect with hereditary ones in important ways. "Children with a family health history of chronic diseases," the CDC's website explains, "can benefit from developing good lifestyle habits, such as exercising and eating healthy, right away. These habits can benefit the entire family and might help prevent or delay these conditions." Lifestyle is about culture, and analyzing culture, as we have seen, is an important part of what historians do. I had seen and feared concrete predispositions in my blood history—an unwavering, inalterable life fate that transcended the conditional relativism of being swept up in history's currents. But what I learned from my family history of illness is that blood history functioned in tandem with lifestyle and environment— that is, the individual choices that I, and members of my family, made. My grandfather made the decision to buy the Cascade farm and reconstruct his own family's yeoman tradition; but he also made the decision to smoke, as did millions of other World War II servicemen, and decades later it cost him his life. In a family history of illness, blood history commingles with individual life choices to determine our past, present, and future.

In other words, clenched in the iron vice of Doig's "blood words" and family genetics are stories of individual choices and even chance happenings—history's fate—expressions of agency, coincidence, serendipity, and just bad luck that lead to the creation of the individual phenotype that becomes you or me. I remain committed to the idea that history mostly happens, rather than is created, but some of it is certainly created by our hands, and this act of making history drove parts of the narrow story that is my family's history. With two decades of university teaching and writing under my belt, I have become far more sympathetic to historians such as Ranke, Collingwood, and others previously discussed, because these forebearers of the discipline researched and narrated examples of a person making history, of conscious choices and individual decisions that shaped events. Ranke might have been interested in Frederick the Great's choices, not my ancestors' decision to homestead in Montana or my grandfather's decision to smoke cigarettes during World War II, but these are still choices. In Ranke's mind, this transcendent moment of cognition, of willful decision making, defines our species, making us uniquely historical beings and in charge of our destinies; but unbeknownst to Ranke, the happenings and coincidences we encounter, and the choices we make, not only create our histories but also create the physical being that becomes us—our bodies are nothing less than historical artifacts, even at the genetic level.

In this manner, I have formulated new questions about the health of the discipline of history while writing this short book. Mainly, has the expansion of the definition of historical agency harmed the discipline and made it less appealing to young people toiling to understand our world and searching for inspiration? When E. P. Thompson, in *The Making of the English Working Class*, argued that the English working class "was present at its own making," did he begin the process of elevating groups of people over individuals, thereby undermining the notion of individual agency in history? When Alfred Crosby, in *Ecological Imperialism*, allowed the smallpox virus and other contagions to become historical agents, demonstrating how they assisted the Western conquest of the globe, what were the consequences for our ability to think that one person alone could alter the fate of the earth, or perhaps just his or her own fate, if a lowly virus could do it, too? When Timothy J. LeCain, in *The Matter of History*, argued that the physical world, from copper molecules and fossil fuels to microorganisms and silk-worms, has directed human civilization in ways beyond our direct control, did that eliminate people from their own history? Finally, if you accept the conclusion reached in this book—that we share the driver's seat of our own lives with diseases and microorganisms—is there even room in my family history of illness for me?

Take this one step further: in today's theoretical paradigms, is there a place for the intriguing counterfactual narrative, such as that of the *Star Trek* episode "City on the Edge of Forever" (1967)? In this story, the peace activist Edith Keeler (played by Joan Collins) is saved by Dr. McCoy when she is supposed to die in a traffic accident. Because she survives, she starts a successful pacifist movement, which forever alters the earth's destiny by delaying the US entry into World War II. As Spock explains to Captain Kirk: "While peace negotiations dragged on, Germany had time to complete its heavy-water experiments" and nuke the United States. As a result, Germany wins the war. In the imagination of Philip K. Dick, in his *The Man in the High Castle*, the US defeat led to the joint occupation of the continental United States by Japan's Pacific States and Germany's Greater Reich.

I am left wondering: are such counterfactuals just the whimsical dreaming of a species that wants to believe that the fate of the world rides on critical decisions made at crucial junctures by key people, maybe even by you or me? Can one person really shape the destiny of the earth with his or her free will when so many other things appear to be in charge of our destiny—our genes, for example, or the microorganisms in our gut? Can one person be historically more influential than copper molecules or silkworms? Historians Jo Guldi and David Armitage would almost certainly answer yes, because, as they have written, "knowledge of the past is . . . a source for understanding the extent to which we have free will in the future." In *The History Manifesto*, they insisted that history has much to offer young people, particularly in a time of metastasizing threats to our democratic institutions and of challenges posed by climate change. Most histories offer "an insistence on free will and the possibility that destiny is unfixed; proof of the power of counterfactual thinking to destabilise the seeming inevitability of current institutions, values, or technologies; and utopian histories about traditions that represent a better world than the one we have now."

But if the answer is "No, they can't outcompete copper molecules and silkworms," then what message, other than sheer intellectual nihilism and political fatalism, does that send to young students of history? Does it discourage them from studying the past and drive them into the conical light of the present, where they yearn for influence over their own lives and therefore choose other fields of study? It reminds me of a refrain from an old Strangers tune: "Whatever happened to the heroes?"

I have come to think that the notion that history simply happens, rather than being created, might contribute indirectly to the widespread ambient "presentism" in today's world, because it takes matters out of our hands and puts them in the hands of an inalterable fate, like genetics or microorganisms. Simultaneously, I have come to think that the way to remedy such ambient presentism is to personalize history a little more, to give back to people the dominant role in their story. Maybe everybody should try the exercise of writing a family history. In a sense, if history just happens, then we are essentially just along for the ride—which, I have concluded, is not true. It is also intellectually unhealthy and not much fun. Indeed, for many today, only the now really matters and history has little to teach. Some historians have speculated that, with climate change and other historically "unprecedented" challenges lurking in the now and the near future, history can provide no roadmaps nor offer precedents for how our species has dealt with similar challenges before. This is because there has never been a similar challenge: the entirety of human history, at least since the emergence of agriculture and writing, has transpired in the Holocene (9,700 BCE) bubble, not the Anthropocene epoch, so rallying the past to explain the here and now—the changing climate and its human consequences, for example, which perhaps will entail massive Southern Hemispheric migrations to the Northern Hemisphere—will become increasingly difficult. Our drama is taking place with the same cast of characters, but in an entirely new theater, one where the air conditioner is broken. I have tried to render my family history of illness as a richly contextualized story, a narrative born of a genuine interest in the deep patterns of the past. But this is a vantage point that many insist is now missing from our world, which is dominated by a fixation on the here and now. It is in personalizing history—showing how it created us, and we created it, and then expanding that story to make broader contextual points about the world—that the power of history can be recovered for many.

The French historian François Hartog identified this ambient "presentism" as beginning with the end of the Cold War; but presentism became more acute after the financial meltdown of 2008, after which the world entered the realm of perpetual "crisis." Our contemporary world, according to Hartog, is characterized by a stagnant present, one bracketed by an unrecognizable past and no real future. Today, he argued, "we live in a world so enslaved to the present that no other viewpoint is considered admissible." He explained that presentism is the "sense that only the present exists, a present characterized at once by the tyranny of the instant and by the treadmill of an unending now." While the "historian practices viewing from afar," the act of creating distance through analytical reflection, today's "rhythms of decision making" conform only to the "tyranny of the immediate." Everything is a crisis that must be acted upon now; there is no slow meditation or careful reflection upon decisions. Certainly, this climate, where "immediacy alone has value," persists in our world.

As I have shown in this book, however, Hartog's observation that "immediacy alone has value" makes for bad medicine, intellectual shallowness, poor self-understanding, and one-dimensional decisions. Take Charles Janeway—the discoverer of "agammaglobulinemia" (today's CVID), whom I discussed earlier—and his lecture "Looking Ahead: The Future of Medicine," a trace of a polymath's philosophy. Before he entered medical school at Cornell University, Janeway had studied "history, economics, social problems and the paths of philosophy and religion" while an undergraduate at Yale University. He studied the cultural influence of Goethe, for example, and understood the importance of medieval European history. These studies in history and culture provided the framework for his global and interdisciplinary medical philosophy, which started with the big bang theory and the "modern condition" and ended with Janeway traveling the globe to heal impoverished children. Janeway situated the body in the broader environment of economics and politics to better understand its ailments.

In 1961, in a short piece titled "A Physician's View of Change," Janeway philosophized about change in this manner: "The modern world, as we know it, is to a large extent the product of science and technology, a world in which the forces of nature are being harnessed to serve the needs of man, and in which, as a result, the necessity is not so much for adaptation to the natural world as to the new world created by human ingenuity," what today's geologists call the Anthropocene epoch. Janeway called on social scientists to study the creation of this world in order to heal people and the planet. "The social and cultural aspects of our environment present a new frontier of knowledge which desperately requires exploration by the scientific method adapted to its peculiarly subtle and difficult problems," he explained. "It is precisely in the formative stage of this new field of the social sciences that imagination and unorthodox thinking are most urgently needed if we are to develop the understanding of individual and group behavior so essential for successful adaptation to our new human environment." On a cautionary note, he continued: "And yet it is precisely in this young field of science, which touches all aspects of human life and its institutions, religion, medicine, law, business, politics, and international relations, that emotion and fear are most readily aroused by the attempt to make objective observations and accurate interpretations of individual and group behavior." To the end, Janeway believed that only by placing the environment and the body in the currents of historical time could medicine really heal life on earth.

On June 18, 1981, Dr. Fred Rosen, also a Harvard pediatrician and immunologist, gave the eulogy at Janeway's service at Harvard's Memorial Church. After the obligatory readings of biblical verses and renditions of choral music by J. S. Bach, Rosen described his friend to the mourning crowd as a "prince of silence," and he dwelt at considerable length on Janeway's "quality of extraordinary intelligence." What made Janeway stand out among his peers? Rosen explained, "There dwelt in him in perfect harmony the two most irreconcilable forces of the Western mind, for he had at once a stern Calvinist asceticism and a deep rational humanism. And in him they found in each other comfort, plausibility and peace." Rosen's observations of Janeway offer a lesson to us all in an age of hyperspecialization in the sciences and of declining support for the arts and humanities at US universities. Let the arts, humanities, and science find "comfort, plausibility and peace" in us all, so that we can find solutions to the challenges we face, and the ones that the earth faces, as Janeway strove to do.

When I presented my draft manuscript to Dr. Vercellotti, who in many regards is not unlike Janeway, he hedged on whether or not I had a family history of illness. "Tough to say," he answered. He suggested we talk by phone about genetics and epigenetics, what he considers to be the key in understanding my CVID diagnosis. I have mentioned epigenetics on several occasions in this book, including in the title of chapter 5, "Phenotypes," and it is an important part of this story. Conrad Waddington, a British biologist, first coined the term *epigenetics* to describe the "mechanisms by which the genes of genotype bring about phenotypic effects." He considered the "relation between phenotypes and genotypes" to be the "kernel of the whole problem of development" in an individual organism. "We certainly need to remember that between genotype and phenotype," he wrote, "there lies a whole complex of developmental processes," and those processes are discerned by the study of epigenetics.

Histone proteins have emerged as the key to understanding Waddington's epigenetic "developmental process." Histone proteins serve as a genetic storage unit, but they do more than just secure the core of DNA. In 1996, David Allis, a molecular biologist, and colleagues began describing the process of "histone modification," whereby chemical change occurs in the histone that modifies the activity of genes without altering their actual sequence. Importantly, when a histone-modified cell divides, it passes the modification down and, hence, reproduces the trait. As Allis explained, "The histone modifications are passed from the parent cell to its daughter cell when cells divide. A cell can thus record 'memory,' and not just for itself but for all its daughter cells." This is how the body's memories, those inscribed onto the body at the genetic level, are passed down through reproduction, and some of those memories can be bad ones and block normal cellular functions, such as antibody secretion. As medical writer Siddhartha Mukherjee said of this process, our "possible selves" in this life are determined by our genes, and histone modifications "conceal some of these selves and reveal others," determining my self rather than other possible selves. Because of these epigenetic forces, a phenotype comes to inhabit "one self among its incipient selves," and this is because of the experiences—because of history. That is, built within our lives are not only historical counterfactuals but also epigenetically determined counterselves, such as one phenotype with CVID, and one without. The "self," Mukherjee wrote, "is suspended between genome and epigenome." This is the "fate" of the individual; but fate is always the product of the times in which we live. Memory proteins—whether B-cells in my immune system, microbial communities in my gut, neuronal forests in my brain, or histones storing my genes—are everywhere in my body. Without them, the body is incapable of adapting and changing and protecting itself, just as without history our species is incapable of remembering, learning, and strengthening our selves and imagining our communities in new ways—a future better than the present.

As mentioned, histone modification can trigger cell changes that damage the body, such as by blocking antibody secretion. This means that an antibody-less self was one of my "possible selves" contained in my genome, and possibly in the genomes of other members of my family as well, and that some idiosyncratic experience—an environmental toxin, or stress while I was department chair—initiated the histone modification that "revealed" the antibody-less me. And what about CVID specifically? As of 2011, genetic studies of CVID have "discovered many novel loci that might underlie the development of CVID," but no single smoking gun. This is because CVID itself is a diverse disease. Researchers have concluded that "CVIDs are a collection of diverse mechanisms leading to complex phenotypes"; and one of those phenotypes is me. I may not fully understand it yet, but I am a product of epigenetic forces and of my genes, my experiences, and my family's experiences—I am history right down to the very genetic fiber of my being.

— · —

Each May, I return to Minneapolis to visit Dr. Vercellotti. His practice is at the Clinics and Surgery Center at the University of Minnesota, a remarkable edifice dedicated to modern medicine, built after my hospitalization. With his colorful bow tie and thick mustache, Dr. Vercellotti is out of place in the corporate atmosphere of the Clinics and Surgery Center. The center is not unlike a giant Verizon store, with flat-screen televisions broadcasting the virtues of clinical trials from every wall and a parade of young service specialists, trained in the intricacies of best practices, greeting patients with tablets as they enter the vast glass atrium. During my visit, Dr. Vercellotti has the lab do a complete blood workup, and he typically looks over the results while I sit impatiently on the examination table.

"Professor Walker, how have you been feeling?" he asks.

"Pretty good," I answer. "How does the blood look?" I ask.

"Fine," he answers.

A painful expression then spreads across his face. He begins fidgeting with the computer mouse because something on the screen has caught his attention. It catches mine, too.

"Is everything okay?" I ask again.

"Yes, I just find it frustrating navigating this new computer system," he replies. "How do you like our new bean-counter's Taj Mahal?" he asks as he swivels in his stool, gesturing at the new Clinics and Surgery Center. The door to the examination room is open, and I see that the sun has poked out from behind the clouds outside, bathing the building in a soft blue light.

"It's pretty amazing," I respond. "But you seem to spend most of your time on the computer."

"Tell me about it," he answers and then begins laughing. "Please take off your shirt."

We then talk campus politics while his hands slide across my neck, up into my armpits, and across my chest, feeling for any swollen or irregular lymph nodes. He looks in my mouth, shines a small light in my eyes, and tests my reflexes. Then, in words that always buoy my spirit, he says, "You need to get out of here, Brett. I actually have sick people that I need to attend to."

With these words, I thank him, leap from my seat, bypass the half dozen checkout specialists requesting a customer satisfaction survey, and charge out of the bean-counter's Taj Mahal into the sun-drenched streets of the East Bank of the University of Minnesota campus. I will do this with Dr. Vercellotti until he retires, and then I will do this with another hematologist or immunologist until I perish, probably of complications from CVID. But that does not matter right now: it has been seven years since my diagnosis, and I am still alive. If anything, my family history has provided me with a sense of optimism about the future; and I am alive because of history—the heroic research of Charles Janeway, the expertise of Dr. Vercellotti, the fabric of my family, and my own experiences.

I return to my home outside Bozeman. LaTrelle and I live on five acres tucked up against the western side of the Bridger Range, not far from the place Ivan Doig originally called home. I am greeted by a little pack of large brown dogs. There is a small orange tractor inside the old barn, and work to do with my hands, which I relish. The vegetables that LaTrelle planted in the garden are starting to sprout, and we hope they survive the inevitable May snowstorms, part of life in the Rocky Mountains. I still have old cars, boats, and motorcycles to tinker with, and it occurs to me once again that, as I connect my past to my present, Doig's "blood words" are about more than simply genetics and predispositions and illnesses. They are about values and priorities and the life rhythms by which we choose to live. My life, and my experience with CVID, may have taken me off the farm, but it certainly has not taken the farm out of me. Neither did it take me out of Big Sky Country. I really had not thought about it, but throughout my life I have continued to rehearse Montana farm life because of the impression it made on me during my birdlike childhood: it was the first thing I laid eyes on. In this way, it was burned into my mind and will always be there, no matter where life takes me. I now see that my character, my values, my intelligence, my toughness, my weaknesses, my harshness, and my compassion were gifts from my family, ones that I have only now discovered through this book, which is a gift far more precious than any genetic predisposition to disease they may or may not have left me.

NOTES

4   *"I dreaded the cold"*: George Orwell, *Homage to Catalonia,* foreword by Adam Hochschild, introduction by Lionel Trilling (Boston: Mariner Books, 2015), 18.

12 *"They guide the construction of our bodies"*: Ed Yong, *I Contain Multitudes: The Microbes within Us and a Grander View of Life* (New York: HarperCollins, 2016), 12.

CHAPTER 1

15 *"words, like the ideas"*: Joan W. Scott, "Gender: A Useful Category of Historical Analysis," *American Historical Review* 91, no. 5 (December 1986): 1053.

16 *field called narrative medicine*: Andrew Solomon, review of *On the Move,* by Oliver Sacks, *New York Times,* May 11, 2015.

16 *"narrative remains essential"*: William Cronon, "A Place for Stories: Nature, History, and Narrative," *Journal of American History* 78, no. 4 (March 1992): 1350, 1374.

16 *"I always wanted to get people's stories"*: "The Q&A: Oliver Sacks, Neurologist," *Economist,* December 7, 2010.

18 *the reality of "being mortal"*: Atul Gawande, *Being Mortal: Medicine and What Matters in the End* (New York: Metropolitan Books, 2014).

18 *life expectancy in the United States*: Jiaquan Xu et al., "Deaths: Final Data for 2013," *National Vital Statistics Reports* 64, no. 2

(February 16, 2016): 1–118, www.cdc.gov/nchs/data/nvsr/nvsr64/
nvsr64_02.pdf; Sherry L. Murphy et al., "Mortality in the United
States, 2014," *NCHS Data Brief* 229 (December 2015): 1–7, www
.cdc.gov/nchs/data/databriefs/db229.pdf; CDC, "National Center
for Health Statistics: Heart Attack," accessed March 19, 2017, www
.cdc.gov/nchs/fastats/heart-disease.htm; CDC, "United States
Cancer Statistics (USCS): 2012 Top Ten Cancers," May 24, 2016,
https://nccd.cdc.gov/uscs/toptencancers.aspx; Donna L. Hoyert,
"75 Years of Mortality in the United States, 1935-2010," *NCHS
Data Brief* 88 (March 2012), www.cdc.gov/nchs/products/databriefs/
db88.htm; American Heart Association, "Family History and
Heart Disease, Stroke," accessed May 24, 2016, www.heart
.org/HEARTORG/Conditions/More/MyHeartandStrokeNews/
Family-History-and-Heart-Disease-Stroke_UCM_442849_Article
.jsp#.VoRQMqvp2lI; American Cancer Society, "Family Cancer
Syndromes," accessed May 24, 2016, www.cancer.org/cancer/
cancercauses/geneticsandcancer/heredity-and-cancer; NIH,
"Autoimmune Diseases," accessed May 24, 2016, www.niaid.nih
.gov/topics/autoimmune/pages/default.aspx. See also Donna
Jackson Nakazawa, *The Autoimmune Epidemic* (New York:
Touchstone, 2009).

19   *"cause persistent suffering"*: Warwick Anderson and Ian R. Mackay,
Intolerant Bodies: A Short History of Autoimmunity (Baltimore,
MD: Johns Hopkins University Press, 2014), 2–6.

20   *primary immunodeficiency disease*: J. M. Boyle and R. H. Buckley,
"Population Prevalence of Diagnosed Primary Immunodeficiency
Diseases in the United States," *Journal of Clinical Immunology* 27
(2007): 497, 499.

20   *"Questions intersecting life"*: Paul Kalanithi, *When Breath Becomes
Air*, foreword by Abraham Verghese (New York: Random House,
2016), 70, 87.

21   *"What matters to us about the past"*: Naomi Oreskes, "Why I Am a
Presentist," *Science in Context* 26, no. 4 (December 2013): 596, 603.

22   *"Unless everything in a man's memory"*: Wallace Stegner, *Wolf Willow: A History, a Story, and a Memory of the Last Plains Frontier*
(New York: Penguin, 1990), 21.

25   *"memory can be considered scenic"* and *"spontaneous, represents
life"*: Dmitri Nikulin, "Introduction: Memory in Recollection of
Itself," in *Memory: A History*, ed. Dmitri Nikulin (Oxford: Oxford
University Press, 2015), 7, 26.

26   *"almost featureless prairie," "quiescent, close to static,"* and *"seem uncorroborated and delusive"*: Stegner, *Wolf Willow*, 4, 7, 15.

28   *"Once Chuang Chou dreamt"*: *Chuang Tzu: Basic Writings*, trans. Burton Watson (New York: Columbia University Press, 1964), 45.

33   *"it was easy then because"*: Ernest Hemingway, *A Moveable Feast* (New York: Scribner, 1964), 12.

34   *"scrollwork or ornamentation"*: Hemingway, *A Moveable Feast*, 12.

34   *"alternative facts"* and *"fake news"*: Elle Hunt, "What Is Fake News? How to Spot It and What You Can Do to Stop It," *Guardian*, December 17, 2016. An advisor to President Donald J. Trump, Kellyanne Conway first used the term *alternative facts* in an interview with *Meet the Press* on January 22, 2017; see Aaron Blake, "Kellyanne Conway Says Donald Trump's Team Had 'Alternative Facts,' Which Pretty Much Says It All," *Washington Post*, January 22, 2017.

36   *"being-in-the-world"* and *"thrownness"*: Martin Heidegger, *Being and Time*, trans. John Macquarrie and Edward Robinson, with a foreword by Taylor Carman (New York: Harper and Row, 1962), 82, 174, 222.

36   *"facticity"*: Heidegger, *Being and Time*, 329.

37   *"the material me"*: C. S. Sherrington, "Cutaneous Sensations," in *Text-Book of Physiology*, ed. E. A. Schäfer (Edinburgh: Young J. Pentland, 1900), 958, 969, 970, 974.

39   *"there are only two kinds of people in the world"*: Hope Jahren, *Lab Girl* (New York: Vintage, 2016), 44.

CHAPTER 2

40   *An absence of immunoglobulins*: Miguel A. Park et al., "Common Variable Immunodeficiency: A New Look at an Old Disease," *Lancet* 372 (2008): 489–502; Sam Ahn and Charlotte Cunningham-Rundles, "Pathogenesis of Common Variable Immunodeficiency," UpToDate, February 2017, www.uptodate.com/contents/pathogenesis-of-common-variable-immunodeficiency.

42   *his injection was probably the first dose of human gamma globulins*: Robert J. Haggerty and Frederick H. Lovejoy Jr., *Charles A. Janeway: Pediatrician to the World's Children* (Boston: Children's Hospital, Harvard Medical School, 2007), 143–44. See also *The Charles Alderson Janeway Medical Service: A Handbook for Patients and Families*, which states in the front matter: "Dr. Janeway was among the first to experiment with the use of gamma globulin, a blood component, for preventing measles and hepatitis. To test

his theories, Dr. Janeway volunteered to be the first person to be
injected with human gamma globulin" (August 17, 1989, MC-7,
Folder 1.13, BCHA). See also the reflections of Dr. Fred Rosen
in "Harvard University: The Memorial Church; A Celebration
of the Life of Charles Alderson Janeway, 1909–1981," Thursday,
June 18, 1981, in which he stated that it was in Cohn's lab where
Janeway "received the first injection ever of Cohn Fraction II or
gamma-globulin with unforeseen and malign consequences. He
survived to perform the classic studies on 'one shot serum sickness'
with Clinton Van Zandt Hawn, just after the war," MC-7, Folder
1.29, BCHA. Finally, the episode is also mentioned in Fred S.
Rosen, "Profiles in Pediatrics II: Charles A. Janeway," *Journal of
Pediatrics* 125 (1994): 167.

45   *Janeway was predisposed to become a doctor*: Haggerty and Lovejoy,
Charles A. Janeway.

45   *"took time out of his busy schedule"*: Charles A. Janeway, "Medicine, Medical Science and Health: The Thayer Lecture in Clinical
Medicine," *Johns Hopkins Medical Journal* 144 (1979): 95.

46   *instilled in Janeway a historical view of medicine*: Charles A.
Janeway, "Looking Ahead: The Future of Medicine by Charles A.
Janeway, M.D., based on the Marshall Woods Lecture at Brown
University on October 28, 1964," MC-7, Folder 1.29, BCHA.

47   *driven to a pub in his Volkswagen microbus*: letter to World-Wide
Automotive Corporation, March 7, 1957, MC-7, Folder 1.25, BCHA.

47   *"A fine way for our elected representatives"*: Charles Janeway to
Chaplain Martyn D. Keeler, June 8, 1945, "Overseas Correspondence Folder," CLM.

47   *"I am particularly concerned"*: Charles Janeway to Hon. Harry S.
Truman, April 19, 1946, MC-7, Folder 1.25, BCHA.

48   *"first step in a long struggle"* and *"monolithic communist conspiracy
for world domination"*: Charles Janeway to President Lyndon B.
Johnson, October 7, 1964; Charles Janeway to President Lyndon B.
Johnson, May 23, 1967, MC-7, Folder 1.24, BCHA.

48   *"have" nations and the "have-not" nations*: Janeway, "Looking
Ahead, MC-7, Folder 1.29, BCHA.

51   *The science of understanding the role of antibodies in the body's
immune system started not with Janeway*: For an overview of Arne
Tiselius's career and contributions, see Frank W. Putnam, "Alpha-,
Beta-, and Gamma-Globulin—Arne Tiselius and the Advent of
Electrophoresis," *Perspectives in Biology and Medicine* 39, no. 3

(Spring 1993): 323–37. On the electrophoresis apparatus itself, see Lily E. Kay, "Laboratory Technology and Biological Knowledge: The Tiselius Electrophoresis Apparatus, 1930–1945," *History and Philosophy of the Life Sciences* 10, no. 1 (1988): 51–72.

51 "*molecular weight of proteins*": The Svedberg and Robin Fåhraeus, "A New Method for the Determination of the Molecular Weight of the Proteins," *Journal of the American Chemical Society* 48, no. 2 (1926): 438.

52 "*I picked out a sample of serum from the refrigerator*": Arne Tiselius, "Reflections from Both Sides of the Counter," *Annual Review of Biochemistry* 37, no. 1 (1968): 6.

52 *Tiselius labeled in descending order of mobility*: Arne Tiselius, "Electrophoresis of Serum Globulin I," *Biochemical Journal* 31, no. 2 (February 1937): 313–17; Arne Tiselius, "Electrophoresis of Serum Globulin II: Electrophoretic Analysis of Normal and Immune Sera," *Biochemical Journal* 31, no. 3 (July 1937): 1466.

52 "*The fastest of these components could be identified with serum albumin*": Arne Tiselius, "A New Apparatus for Electrophoretic Analysis of Colloidal Mixtures," *Transactions of the Faraday Society* 33 (1937): 531. He concluded this paper by explaining, "By suitable compensation the experiment can be arranged so that the different components can be isolated," which is precisely what happened in later research (531). Tiselius named the serum *globulin* in two successive papers: Tiselius, "Electrophoresis of Serum Globulin I," 313–17; Tiselius, "Electrophoresis of Serum Globulin II," 1466.

53 "*relationship of antibodies to these components*": Arne Tiselius and Elvin A. Kabat, "An Electrophoretic Study of Immune Sera and Purified Antibody Preparations," *Journal of Experimental Medicine* 69, no. 1 (January 1939): 119. For a summary of these findings, see Arne Tiselius and Elvin A. Kabat, "Electrophoresis of Immune Serum," *Science*, n.s., 87, no. 2262 (May 1938): 416–17.

53 "*a telegraphic order*": Tiselius, "Reflections from Both Sides of the Counter," 7.

54 "*appeared quite groggy and irrational*," "*safe, stable, compact blood derivative*," and "*all seven patients were given albumin*": John Curling, Neil Goss, and Joseph Bertolini, "The History and Development of the Plasma Protein Fractionation Industry," in *Production of Plasma Proteins for Therapeutic Use*, ed. Joseph Bertolini, Neil Goss, and John Curling (Hoboken, NJ: John Wiley and Sons, 2013), 6–7. See also Raif S. Geha, "Charles A. Janeway and Fred S.

Rosen: The Discovery of Gamma Globulin Therapy and Primary Immunodeficiency Disease at Boston Children's Hospital," *Journal of Allergy and Clinical Immunology* 116, no. 4 (October 2005), 937–40.

55   *"useful and stable concentrates"*: J. L. Oncely et al., "The Separation of the Antibodies, Isoagglutinins, Prothrombin, Plasminogen and β1-Lipoprotein into Subfractions of Human Plasma," *Journal of the American Chemical Society* 71, no. 2 (February 1, 1949): 541–42; H. F. Deutsch, R. A. Alberty, and L. J. Gosting, "Biophysical Studies of Blood Plasma Proteins: IV. Separation and Purification of a New Globulin from Normal Human Plasma," *Journal of Biological Chemistry* 165, no. 1 (September 1, 1946): 35.

55   *"may be of considerable therapeutic value"*: J. Stokes Jr., E. P. Maris, and S. S. Gellis, "Chemical, Clinical, and Immunological Studies on the Products of Human Plasma Fractionation: XI, The Use of Concentrated Normal Human Serum Gamma Globulin (Human Immune Serum Globulin) in the Prophylaxis and Treatment of Measles," *Journal of Clinical Investigation* 23, no. 4 (July 1, 1944): 540.

56   *"This is the form of civilian advisory function," "The control of infectious diseases by passive immunization"*: Edwin J. Cohn, "Blood Proteins and Their Therapeutic Value," *Science*, n.s., 101, no. 2612 (January 19, 1945): 52, 56.

57   *"when you'd take the military out of it"*: Curling, Goss, and Bertolini, "The History and Development of the Plasma Protein Fractionation Industry," 8.

58   *"The plasma fractionation program"*: Charles Janeway to Major George Austin Jr., June 7, 1945, Location 5th Field Hospital, "Overseas Correspondence Folder," CLM.

58   *"it was found last winter," "considerable uniformity of antibody content,"* and *"the pools from which these samples are derived"*: Charles A. Janeway, "Use of Concentrated Human Serum γ-globulin in the Prevention and Attenuation of Measles," *Bulletin of the New York Academy of Medicine* 21, no. 4 (1945): 208.

59   *"absence of serum gamma globulins," "We wish to present an entity," "Although the infections," "One boy had sepsis 18 times,"* and *"It is postulated"*: Ogden C. Bruton et al., "Absence of Serum Gamma Globulin," *American Journal of Diseases of Children* 84, no. 5 (1952): 632–33.

61   *"New disease," "leaves the body of the victim,"* and *"before the days of penicillin"*: William L. Laurence, "Three Physicians Tell of New

Disease, Lack of Gamma Globulin Cuts Resistance to Infection —
Adrenal Study Reported," *New York Times*, May 6, 1953.

62   *"Agammaglobulinemia is a syndrome"*: David Gitlin and Charles A.
Janeway, "Agammaglobulinemia: Congenital, Acquired, and Tran-
sient Forms," in *Progress in Hematology*, ed. Leandro M. Tocantins
(New York: Grune and Stratton, 1956–57), 1:318, 319, 320, 325, 326.

63   *"Many of the families' brothers"* and *"like diabetes"*: David Gitlin
and Charles A. Janeway, "Agammaglobulinemia," *Scientific American* 197, no. 1 (July 1957): 93–105.

CHAPTER 3

66   *"tonalities"*: Vladimir Nabokov, *Speak, Memory: An Autobiography
Revisited* (New York: Vintage, 1989), 170–71.

69   *"In probing my childhood"* and *"sense of time"*: Nabokov, *Speak,
Memory*, 20–21.

70   *"I felt myself plunged"* and *"time's common flow"*: Nabokov, *Speak,
Memory*, 21.

70   *"The act of vividly recalling,"* *"Over the shoulder of my past,"* *"One
is always at home with one's past,"* *"There is, it would seem,"* *"I
witness with pleasure,"* and *"survive captivity"*: Nabokov, *Speak,
Memory*, 75, 82, 116, 166–67, 170–71, 233.

73   *"added to their practices"* and *"When visiting the doctor"*: Rima D.
Apple, *Mothers and Medicine: A Social History of Infant Feeding,
1890–1950* (Madison: University of Wisconsin Press, 1987), 77–78.

75   *"Female breast evoked deep . . . currents of meaning"*: Londa
Schiebinger, *Nature's Body: Gender in the Making of Modern
Science* (Boston: Beacon Press, 1993), 41, 40–74.

77   *Early Europeans used perforated bull's horns*: Ian G. Wickes, "A
History of Infant Feeding: Part I, Primitive Peoples: Ancient Works:
Renaissance Writers," *Archives of Disease in Childhood* 28, no. 138
(April 1953): 151–58; Ian G. Wickes, "A History of Infant Feeding:
Part II, Seventeenth and Eighteenth Centuries," *Archives of Dis-
ease in Childhood* 28, no. 139 (June 1953): 232–40; Ian G. Wickes,
"A History of Infant Feeding: Part III, Eighteenth and Nineteenth
Century Writers," *Archives of Disease in Childhood* 28, no. 140
(August 1953): 332–40; Ian G. Wickes, "A History of Infant Feeding:
Part IV, Nineteenth Century Continued," *Archives of Disease in
Childhood* 28, no. 141 (October 1953): 416–22; Ian G. Wickes, "A
History of Infant Feeding: Part V, Nineteenth Century Concluded
and Twentieth Century," *Archives of Disease in Childhood* 28,

no. 142 (December 1953): 495–502; Samuel X. Radbill, "Infant Feeding through the Ages," *Clinical Pediatrics* 20, no. 10 (1981): 613–21; Thelma E. Patrick, Rita Pickler, and Emily E. Stevens, "A History of Infant Feeding," *Journal of Perinatal Education* 18, no. 2 (Spring 2009): 32–39; and Samuel J. Fomon, "Infant Feeding in the 20th Century: Formula and Beikost," *Journal of Nutrition* 131, no. 2 (February 2001): 409S–420S.

81   *"For the past 14 months"*: Ogden C. Bruton, "Agammaglobulin- emia," *Pediatrics* 9 (1952): 726.

82   *Given the importance of Bruton's tyrosine kinase*: Lea Ann Hansen, "Bruton's Tyrosine Kinase: An Exciting New Target for Treatment of B-Cell Malignancies," Cancer Therapy Advisor, January 12, 2012, www.cancertherapyadvisor.com/hematologic-cancers/brutons -tyrosine-kinase-an-exciting-new-target-for-treatment-of-b-cell -malignancies/article/222861.

84   *Ernest Moro*: Angela Weirich and Georg F. Hoffmann, "Ernst Moro (1874–1951)—a Great Pediatric Career Started at the Rise of University-Based Pediatric Research but Was Curtailed in the Shadows of Nazi Laws," *European Journal of Pediatrics* 164, no. 10 (October 2005): 599–606.

85   *Niels Kaj Jerne*: Thomas Soderqvist, *Science as Autobiography: The Troubled Life of Niels Jerne*, trans. David Mel Paul (New Haven, CT: Yale University Press, 2003).

89   *Marin Terrace School in Mill Valley*: "Marin Terrace School: A Homestead Headlines Article by Chuck Oldenburg," Mill Valley Historical Society, December 3, 2015, www.mvhistory.org/history-of/ history-of-homestead-valley/marin-terrace-school.

91   *"The remembering begins out of that new silence," "Memory is a set of sagas we live by,"* and *"eddying but detailed power"*: Ivan Doig, *This House of Sky: Landscapes of a Western Mind* (New York: Harcourt, 1973), 3, 10, 68.

92   *"If . . . somewhere beneath the blood," "a most queer-lit and shadow- chilled time,"* and *"near-neighborhood of dreams"*: Doig, *This House of Sky*, 10, 106.

92   *"blood words," "I admit the marvel," "like pulses of light,"* and *"This set of sagas, memory"*: Doig, *This House of Sky*, 238, 312.

93   *"School struck me"*: Doig, *This House of Sky*, 16.

94   *"strange cynicism about truth," "permitted us to accept,"* and *"line between fiction"*: Mary Karr, *The Art of Memoir* (New York: Harper- Collins, 2015), 85, 86.

94   *"collective moral machinery"*: Karr, *The Art of Memoir*, 87.
94   *"Sometimes it strikes me"*: Karr, *The Art of Memoir*, 88.

CHAPTER 4

97   *"nurse cleans your skin"*: Hope Jahren, *Lab Girl* (New York: Vintage, 2016), 40.
100   *"exterminating all alpha predators"*: David Quammen, *Monsters of God: The Man-Eating Predator in the Jungles of History and the Mind* (New York: W. W. Norton, 2004), 127.
100   *"It struck me that similar cells," "biopolitical hybrid,"* and *"immunity-as-defense"*: Ed Cohen, *A Body Worth Defending: Immunity, Biopolitics, and the Apotheosis of the Modern Body* (Durham, NC: Duke University Press, 2009), 1, 3.
101   *"modernized body"*: Cohen, *A Body Worth Defending*, 7.
101   *"finance capital, philosophical reflection," "localize human beings,"* and *"grotesque body"*: Cohen, *A Body Worth Defending*, 7.
102   *"talk-story"*: Maxine Hong Kingston, *The Woman Warrior: Memoirs of a Girlhood among Ghosts* (New York: Vintage International, 1989).
108   *"My mother's suffering," "Her life set the emotional tone of my life,"* and *"At the age of twelve"*: Richard Wright, *Black Boy (American Hunger): A Record of Childhood and Youth*, foreword by Edward P. Jones (New York: Harper Perennial Modern Classics, 2006), 100–101.
110   *"since no man ever"*: Thomas Merton, *The Seven Story Mountain: An Autobiography of Faith* (Orlando, FL: Harcourt, 1948), 13.
117   *"Consciousness is a biological process," "human mind and spirituality,"* and *"enormous number"*: Eric R. Kandel, *In Search of Memory: The Emergence of a New Science of the Mind* (New York: W. W. Norton, 2006), 9.
118   *"It gives us a coherent picture," "Without the binding force of memory,"* and *"we would have no awareness"*: Kandel, *In Search of Memory*, 10.
118   *"capacity to live unhistorically," "settle on the threshold,"* and *"chaotic inner world"*: Friedrich Nietzsche, *On the Advantage and Disadvantage of History for Life*, trans. Peter Preuss (Indianapolis, IN: Hackett, 1980), 9.
118   *"History . . . is a nightmare"*: James Joyce, *Ulysses: A Reproduction of the 1922 First Edition* (Mineola, NY: Dover, 2002), 34.
119   *"We must recollect that all of our provisional ideas"*: Sigmund Freud, *On Narcissism: An Introduction* (New York: White Press, 2014).

119   *"vanish if we were already"* and *neuroscience formulated three principles*: Kandel, *In Search of Memory*, 46, 58–67.

120   *"Since the full forest"*: Santiago Ramón y Cajal, "Recollections of My Life," trans. E. Horne Craigie, *Memoirs of the American Philosophical Society* 8, no. 2 (1937): 324.

121   *"plasticity"* and *"permanent functional transformations"*: J. Kornorski, *Conditioned Reflexes and Neuron Organization* (Cambridge: Cambridge University Press, 1948), 79–80.

121   *"I presumed that different forms," "reductionist approach," "learning leads to a change,"* and *"long-term effectiveness of synaptic connections"*: Kandel, *In Search of Memory*, 159–60, 186, 200, 202.

122   *"each human being is brought up"*: Kandel, *In Search of Memory*, 218.

123   *"Almost all of the proteins"* and *"in the brain as in bacteria"*: Kandel, *In Search of Memory*, 236, 264.

123   *"interoception"*: A. D. Craig, "How Do You Feel? Interoception: The Sense of the Physiological Condition of the Body," *Nature Reviews Neuroscience* 3 (August 2002): 655–66; Antonio Damasio, *The Feeling of What Happens: Body and Emotion in the Making of Consciousness* (San Diego, CA: Harcourt Brace, 1999); Elizabeth Johnston and Leah Olson, *The Feeling Brain: The Biology and Psychology of Emotions* (New York: W. W. Norton, 2015).

124   *"wave of bodily disturbance," "perception of the interesting sights or sounds," "the bodily changes follow,"* and *"A purely disembodied human emotion"*: William James, "What Is an Emotion?" *Mind* 9, no. 34 (1884): 189–90, 194, emphasis in the original.

124   *Enteric nervous system, "second brain,"* and *"gut feeling"*: Emeran A. Mayer, "Gut Feelings: The Emerging Biology of Gut-Brain Communication," *Nature Reviews Neuroscience* 12 (August 2011): 453.

124   *"microbiota-gut-brain axis"*: R. M. Stilling, T. G. Dinan, and J. F. Cryan, "Microbial Genes, Brain and Behavior—Epigenetic Regulation of the Gut-Brain Axis," *Genes, Brain and Behavior* 13 (2014): 70.

125   *"interkingdom signaling," "they monitor us,"* and *"we monitor them"*: Mark Lyte, "Microbial Endocrinology in the Microbiome-Gut-Brain Axis: How Bacterial Production and Utilization of Neurochemicals Influence Behavior," *PLOS Pathogens* 9 (November 2013): 1.

125   *microbiological turn in historical studies*: Julia Adeney Thomas, "History and Biology in the Anthropocene: Problems of Scale, Problems of Value," *American Historical Review* 119, no. 5 (2014): 1587–607.

125   *the gut's lymphoid tissue*: Stilling, Dinan, and Cryan, "Microbial Genes, Brain and Behavior," 69.

126   *The body's microbial content*: David Kohn, "When Gut Bacteria Changes Brain Function: Some Researchers Believe That the Microbiome May Play a Role in Regulating How People Think and Feel," *Atlantic*, June 24, 2015. See also Sahar El Aidy, Timothy G. Dinan, and John F. Cryan, "Immune Modulation of the Brain-Gut-Microbe Axis," *Frontiers in Microbiology* 5 (April 2014): 1–4; Rafael Campos-Rodríguez et al., "Stress Modulates Intestinal Secretory Immunoglobulin A," *Frontiers in Integrative Neuroscience* 7 (December 2013): 1–10; John F. Cryan and Timothy G. Dinan, "Mind-Altering Microorganisms: The Impact of the Gut Microbiota on Brain Behavior," *Nature Reviews Neuroscience* 13 (October 2012): 701–12.

127   *BDNF (brain-derived neurotrophic factor) and plasticity*: Kiyofumi Yamada and Toshitaka Nabeshima, "Brain-Derived Neurotrophic Factor/TrkB Signaling in Memory Process," *Journal of Pharmacological Sciences* 91 (2003): 267–70. On serotonin in the "microbiota-gut-brain axis," see S. M. O'Mahony et al., "Serotonin, Tryptophan Metabolism and the Brain-Gut-Microbiome Axis," *Behavioral Brain Research* 277 (January 2015): 32–48. On the "microbiota-gut-brain axis" and autism, see Elaine Y. Hsiao et al., "The Microbiota Modulates Gut Physiology and Behavioral Abnormalities Associated with Autism," *Cell* 155, no. 7 (December 2013): 1451–63.

127   *"happy people tend to be more social"*: Kohn, "When Gut Bacteria Changes Brain Function."

CHAPTER 5

133   *US Centers for Disease Control and Prevention*: CDC, "Fourth National Report on Human Exposure to Environmental Chemicals," February 2015, www.cdc.gov/biomonitoring/pdf/FourthReport_UpdatedTables_Feb2015.pdf.

133   *right chemical trigger*: A. Baccarelli and V. Bollati, "Epigenetics and Environmental Chemicals," *Current Opinion in Pediatrics* 21, no. 2 (April 2009): 243–51; Richard A. Stein, "Epigenetics and Environmental Exposure," *Journal of Epidemiology and Community Health* 66, no. 1 (January 2012): 8–13.

134   *"Memory is essential"*: Eric R. Kandel, *In Search of Memory: The Emergence of a New Science of the Mind* (New York: W. W. Norton, 2006), 10.

134   *key ingredient to the success of societies*: Edward O. Wilson, *The Social Conquest of Earth* (New York: Liveright, 2012).

137   *Francis Bacon . . . dispelled magic, "enlarge knowledge by observation," and "the secrets of nature"*: Quoted in Carolyn Merchant, *The Death of Nature: Women, Ecology, and the Scientific Revolution* (New York: Harper One, 1990), 168–69, 188–89. See also Max Horkheimer and Theodore W. Adorno, *Dialectic of Enlightenment: Philosophical Fragments*, ed. Gunzelin Schmid Noerr; trans. Edmund Jephcott (Stanford, CA: Stanford University Press, 2007).

138   *"No qualities are known which are so occult"*: Quoted in Merchant, *The Death of Nature*, 205.

138   *"God set up mathematical laws in nature"*: Quoted in Merchant, *The Death of Nature*, 205.

138   *"For what is the heart"*: Quoted in Merchant, *The Death of Nature*, 212.

142   *"As it really had been," "archival curiosity," "return to the most pristine sources," "pure perception," "History has been assigned," "I do not deny that I display," and "Nature itself strives to produce form"*: Peter Gay, *Style in History* (New York: Basic Books, 1974), 62, 68–69, 70, 73. See also Leopold von Ranke, *History of the Latin and Teutonic Nations from 1494 to 1514*, trans. Phillip A. Ashworth (White Fish, MT: Kessinger, 2004); and Leonard Krieger, *Ranke: The Meaning of History* (Chicago: University of Chicago Press, 1977), 201.

144   *"As individuals express their life," "Consciousness does not determine life," "When this active life process is presented," "History is nothing but the succession," "circumstances make men just as men," "Men make their own history," and "The tradition of all the dead generations"*: Karl Marx, *Selected Writings*, ed. Lawrence H. Simon (Indianapolis: Hackett, 1994), 107–8, 112, 122, 125, 188.

145   *"How is it possible to get very far"*: Edward P. Thompson, "Under the Same Roof-Tree," *Times Literary Supplement*, May 4, 1973.

145   *"enormous condescension of posterity" and "was present at its own making"*: Edward P. Thompson, *The Making of the English Working Class* (New York: Pantheon, 1963), 12, 9.

146   *The Anglo-Saxon surname Walker*: Mark Antony Lower, *Patronymica Britannica: A Dictionary of the Family Names of the United Kingdom* (London: John Russell Smith, 1860), 370; Charles Wareing Bardsley, *A Dictionary of English and Welsh Surnames*

with Special American Instances (Baltimore, MD: Genealogical Publishing Company, 1968), 789–90.

146   *There is no record of his being knighted*: William A. Shaw, *The Knights of England: A Complete Record from the Earliest Time to the Present Day of the Knights of All the Orders of Chivalry in England, Scotland, and Ireland, and of Knights Bachelors* (London: Central Chancery of the Orders of Knighthood, Sherratt and Hughs, 1906). There is no reference to a Sir William Walker between 1399 and 1424, leading me to believe that he may have been a baronet. Baronetcies appeared in the fourteenth century, so the timing is reasonable.

146   *"territory of the Nausets"*: Simeon L. Deyo, ed., *History of Barnstable County, Massachusetts* (New York: H. W. Blake, 1890), 721–23; Henry C. Kittredge, *Cape Cod: Its People and Their History* (Boston: Houghton Mifflin, 1930); Alice A. Lowe, comp., *Nauset on Cape Cod: A History of Eastham* (Falmouth, MA: Kendall, 1968), 19.

147   *"telling a lye"* and *joining the ranks of New England's governing freemen*: Nathaniel B. Shurtleff, ed., *Records of the Colony of New Plymouth in New England*, vol. 8: *Miscellaneous Records, 1633–1689* (Boston: William White, 1857), 135, 202, 208. See also Enoch Pratt, *A Comprehensive History, Ecclesiastical and Civil, of Eastham, Wellfleet and Orleans, County of Barnstable, Mass. from 1644–1844* (Yarmouth, MA: W. S. Fisher, 1844), 27.

147   *With CVID, what we are looking for is a rare disease*: David Gitlin and Charles A. Janeway, "Agammaglobulinemia," *Scientific American* 197, no. 1 (July 1957): 93–105.

148   *Life expectancies for men in seventeenth-century Europe*: J. P. Griffin, "Changing Life Expectancy throughout History," *Journal of the Royal Society of Medicine* 101, no. 12 (December 2008): 577.

148   *In seventeenth-century Plymouth Colony*: Thomas L. Purvis, *Colonial America to 1763*, ed. Richard Balkin (New York: Facts On File, 1999), 171–77; John Duffy, *Epidemics in Colonial America* (Baton Rouge: Louisiana State University Press, 1971), 104–5, 171–72. See also Oscar Reiss, *Medicine in Colonial America* (Lanham, MD: University Press of America, 2000); and Eric H. Christianson, "Medicine in New England," in *Sickness and Health in America: Readings in the Public History of Medicine and Public Health*, ed. Judith Walzer Leavitt and Ronald L. Numbers (Madison: University of Wisconsin Press, 1978), 47–71.

150 *eruption of Mount Tambora, "The sun, ere he sank," and "a light so angry"*: Gillen D'Arcy Wood, *Tambora: The Eruption That Changed the World* (Princeton, NJ: Princeton University Press, 2014), 174, 183. See also Ian Bostridge, *Schubert's Winter Journey: Anatomy of an Obsession* (New York: Alfred A. Knopf, 2015).

150 *In Ireland a different monster irrupted*: M. R. King, "The Epidemiology of Typhus Fever in Ireland," *Public Health Reports* 42, no. 43 (October 1927): 2643. See also Hugh Fenning, "Typhus Epidemic in Ireland, 1817–1819: Priests, Ministers, Doctors," *Collectanea Hibernica* 41 (1999).

152 *my family began to wash across the continent*: See Ancestry.com records in the bibliography for US Census data related to my family.

153 *He attended Princeton University*: Neal Victor Walker's Princeton University records are held at the Seeley G. Mudd Manuscript Library, Princeton University, "Undergraduate Alumni Records," 1800–1899, http://findingaids.princeton.edu/collections/AC104.02/c10150.

153 *he married and briefly moved to Buffalo*: Per the *Scranton Tribune*, July 27, 1897, 8, "Neal V. Walker, who has been employed in Buffalo for some time, returned Saturday. He and his father, N. L. Walker[,] will go to Keelersburg, where he will assist in managing the lumber business which his father has there." Earlier in 1897, Neal Victor had traveled to Nicholson from Buffalo, New York, to attend New Year's celebrations there. See *Scranton Tribune*, January 2, 1897, 7.

154 *his property in Highland Park went up for auction*: "Treasurer's Sale of Seated and Unseated Lands For Unpaid Taxes in Lackawanna County, Years 1897 and 1898," *Scranton Tribune*, April 24, 1900.

154 *he attended an event at the Elm Park United Methodist Church in Scranton, and his World War I draft card*: Ancestry.com, "Pennsylvania and New Jersey, Church and Town Records, 1708–1985," Historical Society of Pennsylvania, Philadelphia, Pennsylvania, Collection Name: Historic Pennsylvania Church and Town Records, Reel 526, Ancestry.com database, 2011; Ancestry.com, "US City Directories, 1822–1995," Ancestry.com database, 2011; Ancestry.com, "US, World War I Draft Registration Cards, 1917–1918," Registration State: Missouri; Registration County: Lawrence, Roll: 1683399, Ancestry.com database, 2005.

155   *alone and paralyzed in Kansas City*: Ancestry.com, "US, Social
      Security Applications and Claims Index, 1936–2007," Ancestry
      .com database, 2015; Ancestry.com, "Missouri, Death Certificates,
      1910–1962," Ancestry.com database, 2015.

156   *newspaper titled The Menace*: Justin Nordstrom, *Danger on the
      Doorstep: Anti-Catholicism and American Print Culture in the
      Progressive Era* (Notre Dame, IN: University of Notre Dame Press,
      2006). See also Matt Pearce, "A Century Ago, a Popular Missouri
      Newspaper Demonized a Religious Minority: Catholics," *Los
      Angeles Times*, December 9, 2015. My quotes from *The Menace*
      are from front-page stories on May 5, 1912, November 1, 1913, and
      September 5, 1914. I am grateful to Harvard's interlibrary loan staff
      for making *The Menace* available.

158   *importance of culture in determining historical events* and *"indissol-
      uble elements of the material"*: Raymond Williams, *Marxism and
      Literature*, Marxist Introductions series (Oxford: Oxford University
      Press, 1978), 99, 82.

159   *"All knowledge that is about human society"* and *"This is not to say
      that facts"*: Edward W. Said, *Covering Islam: How the Media and
      the Experts Determine How We See the Rest of the World* (New
      York: Pantheon, 1981), 154–56.

160   *"members of even the smallest nation"*: Benedict Anderson,
      *Imagined Communities: Reflections on the Origins and Spread of
      Nationalism* (London: Verso, 1983), 49.

160   *"narrative mode of representation," "its use in any field of study,"*
      and *"discipline that produces narrative"*: Hayden White, "The
      Question of Narrative in Contemporary Historical Theory," *History
      and Theory*, 23, no. 1 (February 1984): 1.

160   *"continued use by historians"*: Hayden White, "The Value of
      Narrativity in the Representation of Reality," in *On Narrative*, ed.
      W. J. T. Mitchell (Chicago: University of Chicago Press, 1981), 4.

161   *"universal structures"* and *"many historical events"*: Michel Fou-
      cault, *The Foucault Reader*, ed. Paul Rabinow (New York: Vintage,
      2010), 46.

162   *"bio-power," "controlled insertion of bodies,"* and *"The perfect disci-
      plinary apparatus"*: Foucault, *The Foucault Reader*, 263, 191–92.

162   *"words, like the ideas"*: Joan W. Scott, "Gender: A Useful Cate-
      gory of Historical Analysis," *American Historical Review* 91, no. 5
      (December 1986): 1053.

163   *EgyptAir Flight 990*: William Langewiesche, "The Crash of Egypt-Air 990," *Atlantic*, November 2001.

CHAPTER 6

170   *With a digital recorder in hand*: Gene and Frances Dwyer, interview by author, Great Falls, MT, October 10, 2014, November 2, 2014, and April 11, 2016. These interviews are part of the author's private collection.

173   *According to the US Centers for Disease Control and Prevention*: CDC, "United States Life Tables, 2003," *National Vital Statistics Reports* 54, no. 14 (April 19, 2006): 26–28, www.cdc.gov/nchs/data/nvsr/nvsr54/nvsr54_14.pdf.

174   *It was an eventful couple of months for the young pair*: Ancestry.com, "Montana, County Marriages, 1865–1950," Ancestry.com database, 2014; Ancestry.com, "Leroy O. Belote in the U.S. World War II Army Enlistment Records, 1938–1946," National Archives and Records Administration, Ancestry.com database, 2014; Ancestry.com, "Leroy Belote in the U.S., Social Security Death Index, 1935–2014," Issue State: Montana; Issue Date: Before 1951; Ancestry.com database, 2011.

176   *served in 1759 in the French and Indian War*: Ancestry.com, "Connecticut Soldiers, French and Indian War, 1755–62," comp. Rose Iris Guertin, Ancestry.com database, 2000.

176   *The Belotes faced their own infectious challenges in the nineteenth-century Midwest*: Walter J. Daly, "The Black Cholera Comes to the Central Valley of America in the 19th Century—1832, 1849, and Later," *Transactions of the American Clinical and Climatological Association* 119 (2008): 143–53.

177   *"pleased Providence to afflict"*: "Public Health in Indiana," special issue, *The Indiana Historian: A Magazine Exploring Indiana History* (March 1998): 5.

178   *germ theory only began to gain traction*: Linda Nash, *Inescapable Ecologies: A History of Environment, Disease, and Knowledge* (Berkeley: University of California Press, 2007); Gregg Mitman, *Breathing Space: How Allergies Shape Our Lives and Landscapes* (New Haven, CT: Yale University Press, 2008).

178   *mysterious "milk sickness"*: William D. Snively, "Discoverer of the Cause of Milk Sickness," *Journal of the American Medical Association* 196, no. 12 (June 20, 1966): 103–8; Walter J. Daly, "The 'Slows': The Torment of Milk Sickness on the Midwest Frontier," *Indiana*

Magazine of History 102 (March 2006): 29–40. On the career of Luther D. Waterman, see "Dr. Luther D. Waterman Dies at 87 Years," *Indianapolis Medical Journal* 21, no. 7 (July 1918): 352–53.

178   *"The testimony adduced"*: Snively, "Discoverer of the Cause of Milk Sickness," 6.

179   *Jefferson M. Belote [and family] spent their lives in the Midwest*: See Ancestry.com records in the bibliography for US Census data related to my family.

179   *pulled up his Midwestern stakes and eventually moved to Montana*: See Ancestry.com records in the bibliography for US Census data related to my family.

180   *the key ingredients for bringing the Belote family to Montana*: Michael P. Malone, Richard B. Roeder, and William L. Lang, *Montana: A History of Two Centuries*, rev. ed. (Seattle: University of Washington Press, 1976), 172–200, 232–42, 280–85.

183   *Then came drought*: M. L. Wilson, "Dry Farming in the North Central Montana 'Triangle,'" *Montana Extension Service Bulletin*, no. 66 (June 1923), 25, 28–29, and 41.

187   *In my first book*: Brett L. Walker, *The Conquest of Ainu Lands: Ecology and Culture in Japanese Expansion, 1590–1800* (Berkeley: University of California Press, 2001).

187   *"autonomous, independent energies"*: Donald Worster, "Transformations of the Earth: Toward an Agroecological Perspective in History," *Journal of American History* 76, no. 4 (March 1990): 1089.

188   *"reenact" and "historical imagination"*: R. G. Collingwood, *The Idea of History*, edited and introduction by Jan Van Der Dussen (Oxford: Oxford University Press, 1994), 209–13.

188   *"we must beware of postulating"*: Marc Bloch, *The Historian's Craft: Reflections on the Nature and Uses of History and the Techniques and Methods of Those Who Write It*, trans. Peter Putnam, introduction by Joseph R. Strayer (New York: Vintage, 1964), 125.

190   *"ordered entities, from molecules to microbes"*: David Christian, *Maps of Time: An Introduction to Big History*, foreword by William H. McNeill (Berkeley: University of California Press, 2004), 26–27.

190   *"has always been there"*: Benoit Mandelbrot, *The Fractalist: Memoir of a Scientific Maverick* (New York: Vintage, 2014), 256. See also Benoit Mandelbrot, "How Long Is the Coast of Britain? Statistical Self-Similarity and Fractional Dimension," *Science*, n.s., 156, no. 3775 (May 5, 1967): 636–38.

191   *"proteins that dominate the chemistry"*: Christian, *Maps of Time*, 96.

191   *"living organisms explore their environment"* and *"deliberately think about the past and imagine the future"*: Christian, *Maps of Time*, 80, 146.

192   *"out there,"* triclosan, and *"Our bodies are environments for the bacteria"*: Edmund Russell, *Evolutionary History: Uniting History and Biology to Understand Life on Earth* (Cambridge: Cambridge University Press, 2011), 5, 31–41, 33.

193   *"point of rupture," "features of culture," "human physiology,"* and *"sameness"*: Daniel Lord Smail, *On Deep History and the Brain* (Berkeley: University of California Press, 2008), 4, 8.

194   *"I do not hold with the idea that a consciousness"*: Smail, *On Deep History and the Brain*, 57.

194   *"superiority of man over all other creatures"* and *"archival and historical medium"*: Guizot quoted in Smail, *On Deep History and the Brain*, 50, 58–59.

195   *"individuals to negotiate," "The existence of brain structures and body chemicals,"* and *"demands that we acknowledge"*: Smail, *On Deep History and the Brain*, 113–14.

195   *"If this age has anything to teach us"*: Timothy J. LeCain, *The Matter of History: How Things Create the Past* (Cambridge: Cambridge University Press, 2017), 326.

196   *"age of coal and steel"*: LeCain, *The Matter of History*, 340.

196   *"much of what makes us so deeply and uniquely human"*: LeCain, *The Matter of History*, 110.

197   *I had asked Benefis Hospitals*: Irene Belote's medical records were not individualized but were instead imbedded in a larger book that encompassed an enormous amount of information about other patients. Record keepers from Benefis Hospitals, which now runs the Great Falls hospital, were kind enough to send me the notations from this book. In addition to LeRoy O. Belote's medical records, I was sent seventeen different records, which ranged from blood tests to "Personal History and Physical Examination" reports. When my grandfather was admitted, Benefis Hospitals was known as Montana Deaconess Hospital Great Falls. See the list of my grandfather's medical records in the bibliography.

EPILOGUE

204   *"My Family Health Portrait"*: CDC, "Document Your Family's Health History," May 8, 2016, www.cdc.gov/Features/Family History.

208   *"merchants of doubt"*: Naomi Oreskes and Erik M. Conway,
       *Merchants of Doubt: How a Handful of Scientists Obscured the
       Truth on Issues from Tobacco Smoke to Global Warming* (New York:
       Bloomsbury Press, 2011).

210   *When E. P. Thompson*: Edward P. Thompson, *The Making of the
       English Working Class* (New York: Pantheon, 1963).

211   *When Alfred Crosby*: Alfred W. Crosby, *The Columbian Exchange:
       Biological and Cultural Consequences of 1492* (Westport, CT:
       Greenwood Press, 1972); Alfred W. Crosby, *Ecological Imperialism:
       The Biological Expansion of Europe, 900–1900* (Cambridge: Cam-
       bridge University Press, 1986).

211   *When Timothy J. LeCain*: Timothy J. LeCain, *The Matter of
       History: How Things Create the Past* (Cambridge: Cambridge
       University Press, 2017).

211   *"City on the Edge of Forever"*: "The City on the Edge of Forever,"
       Star Trek, season 1, episode 28, aired on April 6, 1967, www
       .chakoteya.net/StarTrek/28.htm.

211   *Philip K. Dick*: Philip K. Dick, *The Man in the High Castle* (New
       York: Vintage, 1992).

212   *"Knowledge of the past"*: Jo Guldi and David Armitage, *The History
       Manifesto* (Cambridge: Cambridge University Press, 2014), 31.

212   *"an insistence on free will"*: Guldi and Armitage, *The History Man-
       ifesto*, 30.

213   *Our drama is taking place*: Will Steffen, Paul J. Crutzen, and John
       R. McNeill, "The Anthropocene: Are Humans Now Overwhelm-
       ing the Great Forces of Nature?" *Ambio* 36, no. 8 (December
       2007): 614–21; Dipesh Chakrabarty, "The Climate of History: Four
       Theses," *Critical Inquiry* 35 (Winter 2009): 197–222.

214   *"we live in a world so enslaved to the present"* and *"sense that only
       the present exists"*: François Hartog, *Regimes of Historicity: Pre-
       sentism and Experiences of Time*, trans. Saskia Brown (New York:
       Columbia University Press, 2015), xiii, xiv–xv.

215   *"The modern world"* and *"The social and cultural aspects of our
       environment"*: Charles A. Janeway, "A Physician's View of Change,"
       in *Values and Ideals of American Youth*, ed. Eli Ginzberg, fore-
       word by John W. Gardner (New York: Columbia University Press,
       1961), 17, 20.

216   *"quality of extraordinary intelligence"*: "Harvard University: The Mem-
       orial Church; A Celebration of the Life of Charles Alderson Janeway,
       1909–1981," Thursday, June 18, 1981, MC-7, Folder 1.29, BCHA.

216   *"mechanisms by which the genes"*: C. H. Waddington, "The Epigenotype," *Endeavour* 1 (1942): 18–20.

217   *"histone modifications"*: Siddhartha Mukherjee, "Same but Different: How Epigenetics Can Blur the Line between Nature and Nurture," *New Yorker*, May 2, 2016.

217   *"possible selves," "conceal some of these selves and reveal others,"* and *"is suspended between genome and epigenome"*: Mukherjee, "Same but Different." See also Siddhartha Mukherjee, *The Gene: An Intimate History* (New York: Scribner, 2016).

218   *"CVIDs are a collection of diverse mechanisms"*: Jordon S. Orange et al., "Genome-Wide Association Identifies Diverse Causes of Common Variable Immunodeficiency," *Journal of Allergy and Clinical Immunology* 127, no. 6 (2011): 1360–67.

BIBLIOGRAPHY

ABBREVIATIONS

BCHA Charles Alderson Janeway Papers and Manuscript Collection,
       Boston Children's Hospital Archives
CDC   Centers for Disease Control and Prevention
CLM   Papers of Charles A. Janeway, Rare Books Collection, Count-
       way Library of Medicine, Harvard University
NIH   National Institutes of Health

ARCHIVAL SOURCES

*The Charles Alderson Janeway Medical Service: A Handbook for Patients
   and Families.* August 17, 1989. MC-7, Folder 1.13, BCHA.
Charles Janeway to Chaplain Martyn D. Keeler. June 8, 1945. "Overseas
   Correspondence Folder," CLM.
"Harvard University: The Memorial Church; A Celebration of the Life
   of Charles Alderson Janeway, 1909–1981." Thursday, June 18, 1981.
   MC-7, Folder 1.29, BCHA.
"Hon. Harry S. Truman." April 19, 1946. MC-7, Folder 1.25, BCHA.
"Looking Ahead: The Future of Medicine by Charles A. Janeway, M.D."
   Based on the Marshall Woods Lecture at Brown University on Octo-
   ber 28, 1964. MC-7, Folder 1.29, BCHA.
"Major George Austin, Jr., Location 5th Field Hospital, June 7, 1945."
   Overseas Correspondence Folder, CLM.
"President Lyndon B. Johnson." October 7, 1964. MC-7, Folder 1.24,
   BCHA.

"President Lyndon B. Johnson." May 23, 1967. MC-7, Folder 1.24,
    BCHA.
"World-Wide Automotive Corporation." March 7, 1957. MC-7, Folder
    1.25, BCHA.

MEDICAL RECORDS OF LEROY BELOTE

Benefis Hospitals, Great Falls, MT
    Admission Record (admitting date January 4, 1976)
    Admission Record (admitting date September 16, 1976)
    Admission Record (admitting date September 23, 1976)
    Consultation Report (September 23, 1976)
    Echocardiogram Report (September 27, 1976)
    Personal History and Physical Examination (September 16, 1976)
    Personal History and Physical Examination (September 23, 1976)
    X-Ray Report (September 23, 1976)
    X-Ray Report (September 24, 1976)
    X-Ray Report (September 27, 1976)
    X-Ray Report (September 29, 1976)
    X-Ray Report (September 30, 1976)
    X-Ray Report (October 8, 1976)
    X-Ray Report (October 15, 1976)
    X-Ray Report (October 22, 1976)

INTERVIEWS

Gene and Frances Dwyer. Interview by author, Great Falls, MT, Octo-
    ber 10, 2014, November 2, 2014, April 11, 2016.

OTHER SOURCES

Ahn, Sam, and Charlotte Cunningham-Rundles. "Pathogenesis of
    Common Variable Immunodeficiency." UpToDate, February 2017.
    www.uptodate.com/contents/pathogenesis-of-common-variable
    -immunodeficiency.
American Cancer Society. "Family Cancer Syndromes." Accessed
    May 24, 2016. www.cancer.org/cancer/cancercauses/geneticsand
    cancer/heredity-and-cancer.
American Heart Association. "Family History and Heart Disease, Stroke."
    Accessed May 24, 2016. www.heart.org/HEARTORG/Conditions/
    More/MyHeartandStrokeNews/Family-History-and-Heart-Disease
    -Stroke_UCM_442849_Article.jsp#.VoRQMqvp2lI.

Ancestry.com. "1850 United States Federal Census." Census Place: Gibson, Susquehanna, Pennsylvania. Roll: M432-829. Page: 289A. Image: 573. Ancestry.com database, 2009.

———. "1870 United States Federal Census." Census Place: Salem, Wayne, Pennsylvania. Roll: M593-1464. Page: 267A. Image: 517. Family History Library Film: 552963. Ancestry.com database, 2009.

———. "1880 United States Federal Census." Census Place: Hamilton, Wayne, Pennsylvania. Roll: 1203. Family History Film: 1255203. Page: 307B. Enumeration District: 020. Ancestry.com database, 2010.

———. "1880 United States Federal Census." Census Place: Nicholson, Wyoming, Pennsylvania. Roll: 1205. Family History Film: 1255205. Page: 110B. Enumeration District: 210. Ancestry.com database and Church of Jesus Christ of Latter-day Saints, 2010.

———. "1880 United States Federal Census." Census Place: Van Buren, LaGrange, Indiana. Roll: 290. Family History Film: 1254290. Page: 308D. Enumeration District: 013. Image: 0641. Ancestry.com database and Church of Jesus Christ of Latter-day Saints, 2010.

———. "1900 United States Federal Census." Census Place: Nicholson, Wyoming, Pennsylvania. Roll: 1500. Page: 6B. Enumeration District: 0145. FHL microfilm: 1241500. Ancestry.com database, 2004.

———. "1900 United States Federal Census." Census Place: Olga, Cavalier, North Dakota. Roll: 1227. Page: 15A. Enumeration District: 0048. FHL microfilm: 1241227. Ancestry.com database, 2004.

———. "1900 United States Federal Census." Census Place: South Abington, Lackawanna, Pennsylvania. Roll: 1422. Page: B. Enumeration District: 0117. FHL microfilm: 1241422. Ancestry.com database, 2004.

———. "1910 United States Federal Census." Census Place: Aurora Ward 1, Lawrence, Missouri. Roll: T624-795. Page: 5A. Enumeration District: 0086. FHL microfilm: 1374808. Ancestry.com database, 2006.

———. "1910 United States Federal Census." Census Place: Aurora Ward 3, Lawrence, Missouri. Roll: T624-795. Page: 5B. Enumeration District: 0088. FHL microfilm: 1374808. Ancestry.com database, 2006.

———. "1920 United States Federal Census." Census Place: Angola, Steuben, Indiana. Roll: T625-461. Page: 2B. Enumeration District: 160. Image: 434. Ancestry.com database, 2010.

———. "1920 United States Federal Census." Census Place: Casper Ward 1, Natrona, Wyoming. Roll: T625-932. Page: 12A. Enumeration District: 101. Image: 48. Ancestry.com database, 2010.

———. "1920 United States Federal Census." Census Place: Casper Ward 3, Natrona, Wyoming. Roll: T625-2028. Page: 5B. Enumeration District: 75. Image: 122. Ancestry.com database, 2010.

———. "1920 United States Federal Census." Census Place: Great Falls Ward 4, Cascade, Montana. Roll: T625-968. Page: 2A. Enumeration District: 30. Image: 504. Ancestry.com database, 2010.

———. "1930 United States Federal Census." Census Place: Enderlin, Ransom, North Dakota. Roll: 1741. Page: 7A. Enumeration District: 0009. Image: 71.0. FHL microfilm: 2341475. Ancestry.com database, 2002.

———. "1930 United States Federal Census." Census Place: Kansas City, Jackson, Missouri. Roll: 1198. Page: 6A. Enumeration District: 0131. Image: 381.0. FHL microfilm: 2340933. Ancestry.com database, 2002.

———. "1940 United States Federal Census." Census Place: Casper Ward 3, Natrona, Wyoming. Roll: T627-4573. Page: 62B. Enumeration District: 13-7B. Ancestry.com database, 2010.

———. "1940 United States Federal Census." Census Place: Great Falls, Cascade, Montana. Roll: T627-2214. Page: 4B. Enumeration District: 7-2. Ancestry.com database, 2012.

———. "1940 United States Federal Census." Census Place: Kansas City, Jackson, Missouri. Roll: T627-2165. Page: 83A. Enumeration District: 116-5. Ancestry.com database, 2012.

———. "Connecticut Soldiers, French and Indian War, 1755–62." Compiled by Rose Iris Guertin. Ancestry.com database, 2000.

———. "Leroy Belote in the U.S., Social Security Death Index, 1935–2014." Issue State: Montana. Issue Date: Before 1951. Ancestry.com database, 2011.

———. "Leroy O. Belote in the U.S. World War II Army Enlistment Records, 1938–1946." National Archives and Records Administration. Ancestry.com database, 2014.

———. "Michigan, Marriage Records, 1867–1952." Ancestry.com database, 2015.

———. "Missouri, Death Certificates, 1910–1962." Ancestry.com database, 2015.

———. "Montana, County Marriages, 1865–1950." Ancestry.com database, 2014.

———. "Pennsylvania and New Jersey, Church and Town Records, 1708–1985." Historical Society of Pennsylvania. Philadelphia, Pennsylvania. Collection Name: Historic Pennsylvania Church and Town Records. Reel 526. Ancestry.com database, 2011.

———. "U.S. City Directories, 1822–1995." Ancestry.com database, 2011.

———. "U.S., Social Security Applications and Claims Index, 1936–2007." Ancestry.com database, 2015.

———. "U.S., World War I Draft Registration Cards, 1917–1918." Registration State: Missouri. Registration County: Lawrence. Roll: 1683399. Ancestry.com database, 2005.

———. "U.S., World War I Draft Registration Cards, 1917–1918." Registration State: Montana. Registration County: Chouteau. Roll: 1684107. Ancestry.com database, 2005.

Anderson, Benedict. *Imagined Communities: Reflections on the Origins and Spread of Nationalism.* London: Verso, 1983.

Anderson, Warwick, and Ian R. Mackay. *Intolerant Bodies: A Short History of Autoimmunity.* Baltimore, MD: Johns Hopkins University Press, 2014.

Apple, Rima D. *Mothers and Medicine: A Social History of Infant Feeding, 1890–1950.* Madison: University of Wisconsin Press, 1987.

Baccarelli, A., and V. Bollati. "Epigenetics and Environmental Chemicals." *Current Opinion in Pediatrics* 21, no. 2 (April 2009): 243–51.

Bardsley, Charles Wareing. *A Dictionary of English and Welsh Surnames with Special American Instances.* Baltimore, MD: Genealogical Publishing Company, 1968.

Blake, Aaron. "Kellyanne Conway Says Donald Trump's Team Had 'Alternative Facts,' Which Pretty Much Says It All." *Washington Post*, January 22, 2017.

Bloch, Marc. *The Historian's Craft: Reflections on the Nature and Uses of History and the Techniques and Methods of Those Who Write It.* Translated by Peter Putnam. Introduction by Joseph R. Strayer. New York: Vintage, 1964.

Bostridge, Ian. *Schubert's Winter Journey: Anatomy of an Obsession.* New York: Alfred A. Knopf, 2015.

Boyle, J. M., and R. H. Buckley. "Population Prevalence of Diagnosed Primary Immunodeficiency Diseases in the United States." *Journal of Clinical Immunology* 27 (June 19, 2007): 497–502.

Brownell, James E., Jianxin Zhou, Tamara Ranalli, Ryuji Kobayashi, Diane G. Edmondson, Sharon Y. Roth, and C. David Allis. "Tetrahymena Histone Acetyltransferase A: A Homolog to Yeast Gcn5p Linking Histone Acetylation to Gene Activation." *Cell* 84, no. 6 (March 22, 1996): 843–51.

Bruton, Ogden C. "Agammaglobulinemia." *Pediatrics* 9 (1952): 722–28.

Bruton, Ogden C., Leonard Apt, David Gitlin, and Charles A. Janeway. "Absence of Serum Gamma Globulin." *American Journal of Diseases of Children* 84, no. 5 (1952): 632–36.

Campos-Rodríguez, Rafael, Marycarmen Godinez-Victoria, Edgar Abarca-Rojano, Judith Pacheco-Yepez, Humberto Reyna-Garfias, Reyna Elizabeth Barbosa-Cabrera, and Maria Elisa Drago-Serrano. "Stress Modulates Intestinal Secretory Immunoglobulin A." *Frontiers in Integrative Neuroscience* 7 (December 2013): 1–10.

CDC. "Document Your Family's Health History." Accessed May 8, 2016. www.cdc.gov/Features/FamilyHistory.

———. "Fourth National Report on Human Exposure to Environmental Chemicals." February 2015. www.cdc.gov/biomonitoring/pdf/Fourth Report_UpdatedTables_Feb2015.pdf.

———. "National Center for Health Statistics: Heart Attack." Accessed May 24, 2016. www.cdc.gov/nchs/fastats/heart-disease.htm.

———. "United States Cancer Statistics (USCS): 2012 Top Ten Cancers." Accessed May 24, 2016. https://nccd.cdc.gov/uscs/toptencancers.aspx.

———. "United States Life Tables, 2003." *National Vital Statistics Reports* 54, no. 14 (April 19, 2006): 26–28. www.cdc.gov/nchs/data/nvsr/nvsr54/nvsr54_14.pdf.

Chakrabarty, Dipesh. "The Climate of History: Four Theses." *Critical Inquiry* 35 (Winter 2009): 197–222.

Christian, David. *Maps of Time: An Introduction to Big History*. Foreword by William H. McNeill. Berkeley: University of California Press, 2004.

Christianson, Eric H. "Medicine in New England." In *Sickness and Health in America: Readings in the Public History of Medicine and Public Health,* edited by Judith Walzer Leavitt and Ronald L. Numbers. Madison: University of Wisconsin Press, 1978.

Chuang Tzu: Basic Writings. Translated by Burton Watson. New York: Columbia University Press, 1964.

"City on the Edge of Forever, The." *Star Trek*, season 1, episode 28. Aired on April 6, 1967. www.chakoteya.net/StarTrek/28.htm.

Cohen, Ed. *A Body Worth Defending: Immunity, Biopolitics, and the Apotheosis of the Modern Body*. Durham, NC: Duke University Press, 2009.

Cohn, Edwin J. "Blood Proteins and Their Therapeutic Value." *Science*, n.s., 101, no. 2612 (January 19, 1945): 51–56.

Collingwood, R. G. *The Idea of History*. Edited and introduction by Jan Van Der Dussen. Oxford: Oxford University Press, 1994.

Craig, A. D. "How Do You Feel? Interoception: The Sense of the Physiological Condition of the Body." *Nature Reviews Neuroscience* 3 (August 2002): 655–66.

Cronon, William. "A Place for Stories: Nature, History, and Narrative." *Journal of American History* 78, no. 4 (March 1992): 1347–76.

Crosby, Alfred W. *The Columbian Exchange: Biological and Cultural Consequences of 1492.* Westport, CT: Greenwood Press, 1972.

———. *Ecological Imperialism: The Biological Expansion of Europe, 900–1900.* Cambridge: Cambridge University Press, 1986.

Cryan, John F., and Timothy G. Dinan. "Mind-Altering Microorganisms: The Impact of the Gut Microbiota on Brain Behavior." *Nature Reviews Neuroscience* 13 (October 2012): 701–12.

Curling, John, Neil Goss, and Joseph Bertolini. "The History and Development of the Plasma Protein Fractionation Industry." In *Production of Plasma Proteins for Therapeutic Use,* edited by Joseph Bertolini, Neil Goss, and John Curling. Hoboken, NJ: John Wiley and Sons, 2013.

Daly, Walter J. "The Black Cholera Comes to the Central Valley of America in the 19th Century—1832, 1849, and Later." *Transactions of the American Clinical and Climatological Association* 119 (2008): 143–53.

———. "The 'Slows': The Torment of Milk Sickness on the Midwest Frontier." *Indiana Magazine of History* 102 (March 2006): 29–40.

Damasio, Antonio. *The Feeling of What Happens: Body and Emotion in the Making of Consciousness.* San Diego, CA: Harcourt Brace, 1999.

Deutsch, H. F., R. A. Alberty, and L. J. Gosting. "Biophysical Studies of Blood Plasma Proteins: IV. Separation and Purification of a New Globulin from Normal Human Plasma." *Journal of Biological Chemistry* 165, no. 1 (September 1, 1946): 21–35.

Deyo, Simeon L., ed. *History of Barnstable County, Massachusetts.* New York: H. W. Blake, 1890.

Dick, Philip K. *The Man in the High Castle.* New York: Vintage, 1992.

Doig, Ivan. *This House of Sky: Landscapes of a Western Mind* (New York: Harcourt, 1973.

"Dr. Luther D. Waterman Dies at 87 Years." *Indianapolis Medical Journal* 21, no. 7 (July 1918): 352–53.

Duffy, John. *Epidemics in Colonial America.* Baton Rouge: Louisiana State University Press, 1971.

El Aidy, Sahar, Timothy G. Dinan, and John F. Cryan. "Immune Modulation of the Brain-Gut-Microbe Axis." *Frontiers in Microbiology* 5 (April 2014): 1–4.

Fenning, Hugh. "Typhus Epidemic in Ireland, 1817–1819: Priests, Ministers, Doctors." *Collectanea Hibernica* 41 (1999): 117–52.

Fomon, Samuel J. "Infant Feeding in the 20th Century: Formula and Beikost." *Journal of Nutrition* 131, no. 2 (February 2001): 409S–420S.

Foucault, Michel. *The Foucault Reader*. Edited by Paul Rabinow. New York: Vintage, 2010.

Freud, Sigmund. *On Narcissism: An Introduction*. New York: White Press, 2014.

Gawande, Atul. *Being Mortal: Medicine and What Matters in the End*. New York: Metropolitan, 2014.

Gay, Peter. *Style in History*. New York: Basic Books, 1974.

Geha, Raif S. "Charles A. Janeway and Fred S. Rosen: The Discovery of Gamma Globulin Therapy and Primary Immunodeficiency Disease at Boston Children's Hospital." *Journal of Allergy and Clinical Immunology* 116, no. 4 (October 2005): 937–40.

Gitlin, David, and Charles A. Janeway. "Agammaglobulinemia." *Scientific American* 197, no. 1 (July 1957): 93–105.

———. "Agammaglobulinemia: Congenital, Acquired, and Transient Forms." In *Progress in Hematology*. Vol. 1. Edited by Leandro M. Tocantins. New York: Grune and Stratton, 1956–57.

Griffin, J. P. "Changing Life Expectancy throughout History." *Journal of the Royal Society of Medicine* 101, no. 12 (December 2008): 577.

Guldi, Jo, and David Armitage. *The History Manifesto*. Cambridge: Cambridge University Press, 2014.

Haggerty, Robert J., and Frederick H. Lovejoy Jr. *Charles A. Janeway: Pediatrician to the World's Children*. Boston: Children's Hospital, Harvard Medical School, 2007. Distributed by Harvard University Press.

Hansen, Lea Ann. "Bruton's Tyrosine Kinase: An Exciting New Target for Treatment of B-Cell Malignancies." Cancer Therapy Advisor, January 12, 2012. www.cancertherapyadvisor.com/hematologic -cancers/brutons-tyrosine-kinase-an-exciting-new-target-for-treatment -of-b-cell-malignancies/article/222861.

Hartog, François. *Regimes of Historicity: Presentism and Experiences of Time*. Translated by Saskia Brown. New York: Columbia University Press, 2015.

Heidegger, Martin. *Being and Time*. Translated by John Macquarrie and Edward Robinson. Foreword by Taylor Carman. New York: Harper and Row, 1962.

Hemmingway, Ernest. *A Moveable Feast*. New York: Scribner, 1964.

Horkheimer, Max, and Theodore W. Adorno. *Dialectic of Enlighten-ment: Philosophical Fragments.* Edited by Gunzelin Schmid Noerr. Translated by Edmund Jephcott. Stanford, CA: Stanford University Press, 2007.

Hoyert, Donna L. "75 Years of Mortality in the United States, 1935–2010." *NCHS Data Brief* 88 (March 2012). www.cdc.gov/nchs/products/databriefs/db88.htm.

Hsiao, Elaine Y., et al. "The Microbiota Modulates Gut Physiology and Behavioral Abnormalities Associated with Autism." *Cell* 155, no. 7 (December 2013): 1451–63.

Hunt, Elle. "What Is Fake News? How to Spot It and What You Can Do to Stop It." *Guardian,* December 17, 2016.

Jahren, Hope. *Lab Girl.* New York: Vintage, 2016.

James, William. "What Is an Emotion?" *Mind* 9, no. 34 (1884): 188–205.

Janeway, Charles A. "Medicine, Medical Science and Health: The Thayer Lecture in Clinical Medicine." *Johns Hopkins Medical Journal* 144 (1979): 94–100.

———. "A Physician's View of Change." In *Values and Ideals of American Youth.* Edited by Eli Ginzberg. Foreword by John W. Gardner. New York: Columbia University Press, 1961.

———. "Use of Concentrated Human Serum γ-Globulin in the Prevention and Attenuation of Measles." *Bulletin of the New York Academy of Medicine* 21, no. 4 (1945): 202–22.

Johnston, Elizabeth, and Leah Olson. *The Feeling Brain: The Biology and Psychology of Emotions.* New York: W. W. Norton, 2015.

Joyce, James. *Ulysses: A Reproduction of the 1922 First Edition.* Mineola, NY: Dover, 2002.

Kalanithi, Paul. *When Breath Becomes Air.* Foreword by Abraham Verghese. New York: Random House, 2016.

Kandel, Eric R. *In Search of Memory: The Emergence of a New Science of the Mind.* New York: W. W. Norton, 2006.

Karr, Mary. *The Art of Memoir.* New York: HarperCollins, 2015.

Kay, Lily E. "Laboratory Technology and Biological Knowledge: The Tiselius Electrophoresis Apparatus, 1930–1945." *History and Philosophy of the Life Sciences* 10, no. 1 (1988): 51–72.

King, M. R. "The Epidemiology of Typhus Fever in Ireland." *Public Health Reports* 42, no. 43 (October 1927): 2643.

Kingston, Maxine Hong. *The Woman Warrior: Memoirs of a Girlhood among Ghosts.* New York: Vintage International, 1989.

Kittredge, Henry C. *Cape Cod: Its People and Their History*. Boston: Houghton Mifflin, 1930.

Kohn, David. "When Gut Bacteria Changes Brain Function: Some Researchers Believe That the Microbiome May Play a Role in Regulating How People Think and Feel." *Atlantic*, June 24, 2015.

Kornorski, J. *Conditioned Reflexes and Neuron Organization*. Cambridge: Cambridge University Press, 1948.

Krieger, Leonard. *Ranke: The Meaning of History*. Chicago: University of Chicago Press, 1977.

Langewiesche, William. "The Crash of EgyptAir 990." *Atlantic*, November 2001.

Laurence, William L. "Three Physicians Tell of New Disease, Lack of Gamma Globulin Cuts Resistance to Infection—Adrenal Study Reported." *New York Times*, May 6, 1953.

LeCain, Timothy J. *The Matter of History: How Things Create the Past*. Cambridge: Cambridge University Press, 2017.

Lowe, Alice A., comp. *Nauset on Cape Cod: A History of Eastham*. Falmouth, MA: Kendall, 1968.

Lower, Mark Antony. *Patronymica Britannica: A Dictionary of the Family Names of the United Kingdom*. London: John Russell Smith, 1860.

Lyte, Mark. "Microbial Endocrinology in the Microbiome-Gut-Brain Axis: How Bacterial Production and Utilization of Neurochemicals Influence Behavior." *PLOS Pathogens* 9 (November 2013): 1–4.

Malone, Michael P., Richard B. Roeder, and William L. Lang. *Montana: A History of Two Centuries*, rev. ed. Seattle: University of Washington Press, 1976.

Mandelbrot, Benoit. *The Fractalist: Memoir of a Scientific Maverick*. New York: Vintage, 2014.

———. "How Long Is the Coast of Britain? Statistical Self-Similarity and Fractional Dimension." *Science*, n.s., 156, no. 3775 (May 5, 1967): 636–38.

"Marin Terrace School: A Homestead Headlines Article by Chuck Oldenburg." Mill Valley Historical Society. Accessed December 3, 2015. www.mvhistory.org/history-of/history-of-homestead-valley/marin-terrace-school.

Marx, Karl. *Selected Writings*. Edited by Lawrence H. Simon. Indianapolis: Hackett, 1994.

Mayer, Emeran A. "Gut Feelings: The Emerging Biology of Gut-Brain Communication." *Nature Reviews Neuroscience* 12 (August 2011): 453–66.

The Menace, Aurora, MO, April 15, 1911–20. Library of Congress. http://
chroniclingamerica.loc.gov/lccn/sn88084144.

Merchant, Carolyn. *The Death of Nature: Women, Ecology, and the
Scientific Revolution.* New York: Harper One, 1990.

Merton, Thomas. *The Seven Story Mountain: An Autobiography of Faith.*
Orlando, FL: Harcourt, 1948.

Mitman, Gregg. *Breathing Space: How Allergies Shape Our Lives and
Landscapes.* New Haven, CT: Yale University Press, 2008.

Mukherjee, Siddhartha. *The Gene: An Intimate History.* New York:
Scribner, 2016.

———. "Same but Different: How Epigenetics Can Blur the Line
between Nature and Nurture." *New Yorker,* May 2, 2016.

Murphy, Sherry L., Kenneth D. Kochanek, Jiaquan Xu, and Elizabeth Arias. "Mortality in the United States, 2014." *NCHS Data
Brief* 229 (December 2015): 1–7. www.cdc.gov/nchs/data/databriefs/
db229.pdf.

Nabokov, Vladimir. *Speak, Memory: An Autobiography Revisited.* New
York: Vintage, 1989.

Nakazawa, Donna Jackson. *The Autoimmune Epidemic.* New York:
Touchstone, 2009.

Nash, Linda. *Inescapable Ecologies: A History of Environment, Disease,
and Knowledge.* Berkeley: University of California Press, 2007.

National Cancer Institute, "Types of Treatment." Accessed May 24, 2016.
www.cancer.gov/about-cancer/treatment/types.

Nietzsche, Friedrich. *On the Advantage and Disadvantage of History for
Life.* Translated by Peter Preuss. Indianapolis, IN: Hackett, 1980.

NIH. "Autoimmune Diseases." Accessed May 24, 2016. www.niaid.nih.
gov/topics/autoimmune/pages/default.aspx.

Nikulin, Dmitri. "Introduction: Memory in Recollection of Itself." In
Memory: A History, edited by Dmitri Nikulin. Oxford: Oxford University Press, 2015.

Nordstrom, Justin. *Danger on the Doorstep: Anti-Catholicism and American Print Culture in the Progressive Era.* Notre Dame, IN: University
of Notre Dame Press, 2006.

O'Mahony, S. M., G. Clarke, Y. E. Borre, T. G. Dinan, and J. F. Cryan.
"Serotonin, Tryptophan Metabolism and the Brain-Gut-Microbiome
Axis." *Behavioral Brain Research* 277 (January 2015): 32–48.

Oncely, J. L., M. Melin, D. A. Richert, J. W. Cameron, and P. M. Gross
Jr. "The Separation of the Antibodies, Isoagglutinins, Prothrombin,
Plasminogen and β1-Lipoprotein into Subfractions of Human

Plasma." *Journal of the American Chemical Society* 71, no. 2 (February 1, 1949): 541–50.

Orange, Jordon S., et al. "Genome-Wide Association Identifies Diverse Causes of Common Variable Immunodeficiency." *Journal of Allergy and Clinical Immunology* 127, no. 6 (2011): 1360–67.

Oreskes, Naomi. "Why I Am a Presentist." *Science in Context* 26, no. 4 (December 2013): 595–609.

Oreskes, Naomi, and Erik M. Conway. *Merchants of Doubt: How a Handful of Scientists Obscured the Truth on Issues from Tobacco Smoke to Global Warming*. New York: Bloomsbury Press, 2011.

Orwell, George. *Homage to Catalonia*. Foreword by Adam Hochschild. Introduction by Lionel Trilling. Boston: Mariner, 2015.

Park, Miguel A., James T. Li, John B. Hagan, Daniel E. Maddox, and Roshini S. Abraham. "Common Variable Immunodeficiency: A New Look at an Old Disease." *Lancet* 372 (2008): 489–502.

Patrick, Thelma E., Rita Pickler, and Emily E. Stevens. "A History of Infant Feeding." *Journal of Perinatal Education* 18, no. 2 (Spring 2009): 32–39.

Pearce, Matt. "A Century Ago, a Popular Missouri Newspaper Demonized a Religious Minority: Catholics." *Los Angeles Times*, December 9, 2015.

Pratt, Enoch. *A Comprehensive History, Ecclesiastical and Civil, of Eastham, Wellfleet and Orleans, County of Barnstable, Mass. from 1644–1844*. Yarmouth, MA: W. BS. Fisher, 1844.

"Public Health in Indiana." Special issue, *Indiana Historian: A Magazine Exploring Indiana History* (March 1998): 2–15.

Purvis, Thomas L. *Colonial America to 1763*. Edited by Richard Balkin. New York: Facts On File, 1999.

Putnam, Frank W. "Alpha-, Beta-, and Gamma-Globulin—Arne Tiselius and the Advent of Electrophoresis." *Perspectives in Biology and Medicine* 39, no. 3 (Spring 1993): 323–37.

Quammen, David. *Monsters of God: The Man-Eating Predator in the Jungles of History and the Mind*. New York: W. W. Norton, 2004.

Radbill, Samuel X. "Infant Feeding through the Ages." *Clinical Pediatrics* 20, no. 10 (1981): 613–21.

Ramón y Cajal, Santiago. "Recollections of My Life." Translated by E. Horne Craigie. *Memoirs of the American Philosophical Society* 8, no. 2 (1937).

Ranke, Leopold von. *History of the Latin and Teutonic Nations from 1494 to 1514*. Translated by Phillip A. Ashworth. White Fish, MT: Kessinger, 2004.

Reiss, Oscar. *Medicine in Colonial America*. Lanham, MD: University Press of America, 2000.

Rosen, Fred S. "Profiles in Pediatrics II: Charles A. Janeway." *Journal of Pediatrics* 125 (1994): 167–68.

Russell, Edmund. *Evolutionary History: Uniting History and Biology to Understand Life on Earth*. Cambridge: Cambridge University Press, 2011.

Said, Edward W. *Covering Islam: How the Media and the Experts Determine How We See the Rest of the World*. New York: Pantheon, 1981.

Schiebinger, Londa. *Nature's Body: Gender in the Making of Modern Science*. Boston: Beacon Press, 1993.

Scott, Joan W. "Gender: A Useful Category of Historical Analysis." *American Historical Review* 91, no. 5 (December 1986): 1053–75.

Seeley G. Mudd Manuscript Library, Princeton University. "Undergraduate Alumni Records." 1800–1899. http://findingaids.princeton.edu/collections/AC104.02/c10150.

Shaw, William A. *The Knights of England: A Complete Record from the Earliest Time to the Present Day of the Knights of All the Orders of Chivalry in England, Scotland, and Ireland, and of Knights Bachelors*. London: Central Chancery of the Orders of Knighthood, Sherratt and Hughs, 1906.

Sherrington, C. S. "Cutaneous Sensations." In *Text-Book of Physiology*, edited by E. A. Schäfer. Edinburgh: Young J. Pentland, 1900.

Shurtleff, Nathaniel B., ed. *Records of the Colony of New Plymouth in New England*. Vol. 8: *Miscellaneous Records, 1633–1689*. Boston: William White, 1857.

Smail, Daniel Lord. *On Deep History and the Brain*. Berkeley: University of California Press, 2008.

Snively, William D. "Discoverer of the Cause of Milk Sickness." *Journal of the American Medical Association* 196, no. 12 (June 20, 1966): 103–8.

Soderqvist, Thomas. *Science as Autobiography: The Troubled Life of Niels Jerne*. Translated by David Mel Paul. New Haven, CT: Yale University Press, 2003.

Solomon, Andrew. Review of *On the Move*, by Oliver Sacks. *New York Times*, May 11, 2015.

Steffen, Will, Paul J. Crutzen, and John R. McNeill. "The Anthropocene: Are Humans Now Overwhelming the Great Forces of Nature?" *Ambio* 36, no. 8 (December 2007): 614–21.

Stegner, Wallace. *Wolf Willow: A History, a Story, and a Memory of the Last Plains Frontier*. New York: Penguin, 1990.

Stein, Richard A. "Epigenetics and Environmental Exposure." *Journal of Epidemiology and Community Health* 66, no. 1 (January 2012): 8–13.

Stilling, R. M., T. G. Dinan, and J. F. Cryan. "Microbial Genes, Brain and Behavior—Epigenetic Regulation of the Gut-Brain Axis." *Genes, Brain and Behavior* 13 (2014): 69–86.

Stokes, J., Jr., E. P. Maris, and S. S. Gellis. "Chemical, Clinical, and Immunological Studies on the Products of Human Plasma Fractionation: XI. The Use of Concentrated Normal Human Serum Gamma Globulin (Human Immune Serum Globulin) in the Prophylaxis and Treatment of Measles." *Journal of Clinical Investigation* 23, no. 4 (July 1, 1944): 531–40.

Svedberg, The, and Robin Fåhraeus. "A New Method for the Determination of the Molecular Weight of the Proteins." *Journal of the American Chemical Society* 48, no. 2 (1926): 430–38.

Thomas Adeney, Julia. "History and Biology in the Anthropocene: Problems of Scale, Problems of Value." *American Historical Review* 119, no. 5 (2014): 1587–1607.

Thompson, Edward P. *The Making of the English Working Class*. New York: Pantheon, 1963.

———. "Under the Same Roof-Tree." *Times Literary Supplement*, May 4, 1973.

Tiselius, Arne. "Electrophoresis of Serum Globulin I." *Biochemical Journal* 31, no. 2 (February 1937): 313–17.

———. "Electrophoresis of Serum Globulin II: Electrophoretic Analysis of Normal and Immune Sera." *Biochemical Journal* 31, no. 3 (July 1937): 1464–77.

———. "A New Apparatus for Electrophoretic Analysis of Colloidal Mixtures." *Transactions of the Faraday Society* 33 (1937): 524–31.

———. "Reflections from Both Sides of the Counter." *Annual Review of Biochemistry* 37, no. 1 (1968): 1–23.

Tiselius, Arne, and Elvin A. Kabat. "Electrophoresis of Immune Serum." *Science*, n.s., 87, no. 2262 (May 1938): 416–17.

———. "An Electrophoretic Study of Immune Sera and Purified Antibody Preparations." *Journal of Experimental Medicine* 69, no. 1 (January 1939): 119–31.

Waddington, C. H. "The Epigenotype." *Endeavour* 1 (1942): 18–20.

Walker, Brett L. *The Conquest of Ainu Lands: Ecology and Culture in Japanese Expansion, 1590–1800*. Berkeley: University of California Press, 2001.

———. "Idainaru shûren: Nihon ni okeru shizen kankyô no hakken." In *Nihon no shisô: Shizen to jin'i*, vol. 4. Edited by Karube Tadashi, Kurozumi Makoto, Satô Hirô, and Sueki Fumihiko. Tokyo: Iwanami Koza, 2013.

———. *The Lost Wolves of Japan*. Foreword by William Cronon. Seattle: University of Washington Press, 2005.

———. *Toxic Archipelago: A History of Industrial Disease in Japan*. Foreword by William Cronon. Seattle: University of Washington Press, 2010.

Weirich, Angela, and Georg F. Hoffmann. "Ernst Moro (1874–1951)—a Great Pediatric Career Started at the Rise of University-Based Pediatric Research but Was Curtailed in the Shadows of Nazi Laws." *European Journal of Pediatrics* 164, no. 10 (October 2005): 599–606.

White, Hayden. "The Question of Narrative in Contemporary Historical Theory." *History and Theory* 23, no. 1 (February 1984): 1–33.

———. "The Value of Narrativity in the Representation of Reality." In *On Narrative*. Edited by W. J. T. Mitchell. Chicago: University of Chicago Press, 1981.

Wickes, Ian G. "A History of Infant Feeding: Part I. Primitive Peoples: Ancient Works: Renaissance Writers." *Archives of Disease in Childhood* 28, no. 138 (April 1953): 151–58.

———. "A History of Infant Feeding: Part II. Seventeenth and Eighteenth Centuries." *Archives of Disease in Childhood* 28, no. 139 (June 1953): 232–40.

———. "A History of Infant Feeding: Part III. Eighteenth and Nineteenth Century Writers." *Archives of Disease in Childhood* 28, no. 140 (August 1953): 332–40.

———. "A History of Infant Feeding: Part IV. Nineteenth Century Continued." *Archives of Disease in Childhood* 28, no. 141 (October 1953): 416–22.

———. "A History of Infant Feeding: Part V. Nineteenth Century Concluded and Twentieth Century." *Archives of Disease in Childhood* 28, no. 142 (December 1953): 495–502.

Williams, Raymond. *Marxism and Literature*. Marxist Introductions series. Oxford: Oxford University Press, 1978.

Wilson, Edward O. *The Social Conquest of Earth*. New York: Liveright, 2012.

Wilson, M. L. "Dry Farming in the North Central Montana 'Triangle.'" *Montana Extension Service Bulletin*, no. 66 (June 1923): 1–132.

Wood, Gillen D'Arcy. *Tambora: The Eruption That Changed the World*. Princeton, NJ: Princeton University Press, 2014.

Worster, Donald. "Transformations of the Earth: Toward an Agro-ecological Perspective in History." *Journal of American History* 76, no. 4 (March 1990): 1087–106.

Wright, Richard. *Black Boy (American Hunger): A Record of Childhood and Youth*. Foreword by Edward P. Jones. New York: Harper Perennial Modern Classics, 2006.

Xu, Jiaquan, Sherry L. Murphy, Kenneth D. Kochanek, and Brigham A. Bastian. "Deaths: Final Data for 2013." *National Vital Statistics Reports* 64, no. 2 (February 16, 2016): 1–118. www.cdc.gov/nchs/data/nvsr/nvsr64/nvsr64_02.pdf.

Yamada, Kiyofumi, and Toshitaka Nabeshima. "Brain-Derived Neurotrophic Factor/TrkB Signaling in Memory Process." *Journal of Pharmacological Sciences* 91 (2003): 267–70.

Yong, Ed. *I Contain Multitudes: The Microbes within Us and a Grander View of Life*. New York: HarperCollins, 2016.

INDEX

acquired CVID, 63–64. *See also*
  CVID
adaptive immune system, 80. *See
  also* immune system
Affordable Care Act
  ("Obamacare"), 38
agammaglobulinemia. *See* CVID
agency, historical, 188–89, 210–13
agranulocytosis, 197–98
albumin, 52, 54–55. *See also* blood
  fractionation
Allaire, F. J., 199–202
Allis, David, 217
alpha-globulins, 52–53, 86
"alternative facts," 34
American Association of Blood
  Banks, 56
American Red Cross, 56
Anderson, Benedict, 160
Anderson, Warwick, 19
anorexia, 200
Anthropocene, 50–51, 195–96, 215

antibacterial soaps, 192
antibiotic-resistant bugs, 192, 193
antibodies: in breast milk, 86;
  defined, 40; in immune system,
  83; linked with gammaglobu-
  lins, 53; Tiselius and Svedberg's work on, 51–54. *See also*
  immunoglobulins
antigens, 85
anxiety, 103–4
Apt, Leonard, 59, 80
archives, 166–70
Armitage, David, 212
Aurora, Missouri, 154–58
autism spectrum disorders, 126
autoimmune diseases, 19–20

Bacon, Francis, 137, 138, 142
bacteria: antibiotic-resistant, 192,
  193; bacterial invasion, 59–62,
  82–83, 100
Bacteroides fragilis, 126

white snakeroot, 178–79
Williams, Raymond, 158–59
Wilson, M. L., 184
World War II and war effort, 41–42,
    54–57
Worster, Donald, 187–88, 193, 194.
    See also environmental history
Wright, Richard, 108–9

X-linked agammaglobulinemia
    (Bruton's syndrome), 80–82

Yale University, 185–86
"year without a summer"
    (1815), 150–51, 167–68, 207.
    See also Tambora (Mount)
    eruption
Yong, Ed, 12
Yosemite Valley, California, 69
Your Baby's Health Book (Mead
    Johnson and Co.), 73–74

Zhuangzi, 28–29